TABLE OF CONTENTS

Top 20 Test Taking Tips

1. Carefully follow all the test registration procedures
2. Know the test directions, duration, topics, question types, how many questions
3. Setup a flexible study schedule at least 3-4 weeks before test day
4. Study during the time of day you are most alert, relaxed, and stress free
5. Maximize your learning style; visual learner use visual study aids, auditory learner use auditory study aids
6. Focus on your weakest knowledge base
7. Find a study partner to review with and help clarify questions
8. Practice, practice, practice
9. Get a good night's sleep; don't try to cram the night before the test
10. Eat a well balanced meal
11. Know the exact physical location of the testing site; drive the route to the site prior to test day
12. Bring a set of ear plugs; the testing center could be noisy
13. Wear comfortable, loose fitting, layered clothing to the testing center; prepare for it to be either cold or hot during the test
14. Bring at least 2 current forms of ID to the testing center
15. Arrive to the test early; be prepared to wait and be patient
16. Eliminate the obviously wrong answer choices, then guess the first remaining choice
17. Pace yourself; don't rush, but keep working and move on if you get stuck
18. Maintain a positive attitude even if the test is going poorly
19. Keep your first answer unless you are positive it is wrong
20. Check your work, don't make a careless mistake

Patient Problems

Cardiothoracic Surgery

Cardiac dysrhythmias

Cardiac dysrhythmias, abnormal heart beats, in adults are frequently the result of damage to the conduction system during major cardiac surgery or as the result of a myocardial infarction.

Bradydysrhythmia

Bradydysrhythmias are pulse rates that are abnormally slow.

Complete atrioventricular block may be congenital or a response to surgical trauma.

Sinus bradycardia may be caused by the autonomic nervous system or a response to hypotension and a decrease in oxygenation.

Junctional/nodal rhythms often occur in postsurgical patients when the absence of the P wave is noted, but heart rate and output usually remain stable; unless there is compromise, no treatment is necessary.

Tachydysrhythmia

Tachydysrhythmias are pulse rates that are abnormally fast.

Sinus tachycardia is often caused by illness, such as fever or infection.

Supraventricular tachycardia (200–300 bpm) may have a sudden onset and result in congestive heart failure.

Conduction irregularities

Conduction irregularities are irregular pulses that often occur postoperatively and are usually not significant.

Premature contractions may arise from the atria or ventricles.

SB

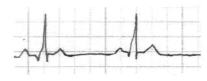 Sinus bradycardia (SB) is caused by a decreased rate of impulse from the sinus node. The pulse and electrocardiogram usually appear normal except for a slower rate. SB is characterized by a regular pulse less than 50–60 bpm with P waves in front of QRS, which are usually normal in shape and duration. The PR interval is 0.12–0.20 seconds; the QRS interval is 0.04–0.11 seconds; and the P:QRS ratio is 1:1.

A number of factors may cause SB:
- Conditions that lower the body's metabolic needs, such as hypothermia or sleep
- Hypotension and a decrease in oxygenation
- Medications, such as calcium channel blockers and β-blockers
- Vagal stimulation that may result from vomiting, suctioning, or defecating
- Increased intracranial pressure
- Myocardial infarction

Treatment involves eliminating the cause, if possible, such as changing medications. Atropine, 0.5–1.0 mg, may be given intravenously to block vagal stimulation. Postoperatively, a pacemaker is inserted for atrial or atrioventricular pacing as well as catecholamine infusion.

ST

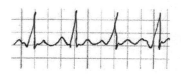

Sinus tachycardia (ST) occurs when the sinus node impulse increases in frequency. ST is characterized by a regular pulse over 100 bpm with P waves before QRS but sometimes part of the preceding T wave. QRS is usually of normal shape and duration (0.04–0.11 seconds) but may have consistent irregularity. The PR interval is 0.12–0.20 seconds, and the P:QRS ratio is 1:1. The rapid pulse decreases diastolic filling time and causes reduced cardiac output with resultant hypotension. Acute pulmonary edema may result from the decreased ventricular filling if untreated.

ST may be caused by a number of factors:
- Acute blood loss
- shock, hypovolemia, and anemia
- Sinus arrhythmia and hypovolemic heart failure
- Hypermetabolic conditions, fever, and infection
- Exertion/ exercise and anxiety
- Medications, such as sympathomimetic drugs

Treatment includes eliminating precipitating factors. With normal left ventricular function, treatment is usually not necessary. Calcium channel blockers and β-blockers may be used to reduce heart rate.

SVT

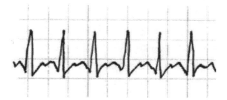

Supraventricular tachycardia (SVT) (> 100 bpm) may have a sudden onset and result in congestive heart failure. Heart rate may increase to 200–300 bpm. SVT originates in the atria rather than the ventricles but is controlled by the tissue in the area of the atrioventricular node rather than the sinoatrial node. Rhythm is usually rapid but regular. The P wave is present but may not be clearly defined as it may be obscured by the preceding T wave, and the QRS complex appears normal. The PR interval is 0.12–0.20 seconds, and the QRS interval is 0.04–0.11 seconds with a P:QRS ratio of 1:1. SVT may be episodic with periods of normal heart rate and rhythm between episodes of SVT, so it is often referred to as paroxysmal SVT. Treatment includes adenosine but may require atrial overdrive pacing or cardioversion. Other medications include verapamil/diltiazem, β-blockers, and digoxin.

SA

Sinus arrhythmia (SA) results from irregular impulses from the sinus node, often paradoxical (increasing with inspiration and decreasing with expiration) because of stimulation of the vagal nerve during inspiration; it rarely causes a negative hemodynamic effect. These cyclic changes in the pulse during respiration are quite common in both children and young adults; they often lessen with age but may persist in some adults. Sinus arrhythmia can, in some cases, relate to heart or valvular disease and may be increased with vagal stimulation for suctioning, vomiting, or defecating. Characteristics of SA include a regular pulse of 50–100 bpm, P waves in front of QRS with a duration of 0.4–0.11 seconds, and a normal shape of QRS, a PR interval of 0.12–0.20 seconds, and a P:QRS ratio of 1:1. Treatment is not necessary unless SA is associated with bradycardia.

PACs

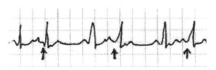

There are three primary types of atrial dysrhythmias, including premature atrial contractions (PACs), atrial flutter, and atrial fibrillation. PACs are essentially extra beats precipitated by an electrical impulse to the atrium before the sinus node impulse. The extra beat may be caused by alcohol, caffeine, nicotine, hypervolemia, hypokalemia, hypermetabolic conditions, atrial ischemia, or infarction. PACs increase the risk of atrial tachyarrhythmias. Characteristics include an irregular pulse because of extra P waves, usually a normal shape and duration of QRS (0.04–0.11 seconds) but QRS may also be abnormal, a PR interval between 0.12–0.20 seconds, and a P:QRS ratio of 1:1. Rhythm is irregular with varying P-P and R-R intervals. PACs can occur in an essentially healthy heart and are not usually cause for concern unless they occur for more than 6 hours and cause severe palpitations. In that case, atrial fibrillation should be suspected. Postsurgical treatment may include atrial pacing, magnesium sulfate, β-blockers, calcium channel blockers, and amiodarone.

AF

Atrial flutter (AF) occurs when the atrial rate is faster, usually 250–400 bpm, than the atrioventricular (AV) node conduction rate so not all of the beats are conducted into the ventricles, effectively blocked at the AV node, preventing ventricular fibrillation although some extra ventricular impulses may go through. AF is caused by the same conditions that cause atrial fibrillation: coronary artery disease, valvular disease, pulmonary disease, heavy alcohol ingestion, and cardiac surgery. AF is characterized by atrial rates of 250–400 bpm with ventricular rates of 75–150 bpm, with a regular ventricular rate. P waves are saw-toothed (referred to as F waves); the shape and duration (0.4–0.11 seconds) of QRS are usually normal; the PR interval may be hard to calculate because of F waves; and the P:QRS ratio is 2–4:1. Symptoms include chest pain, dyspnea, and hypotension. Treatment includes the following: Rapid atrial pacing, Cardioversion if the condition is unstable, Medications to slow ventricular rate and conduction through the AV node, such as Cardizem (Diltiazem) and verapamil (Calan), Medications to convert to sinus rhythm, such as ibutilide (Corvert), quinidine (Cardioquin), disopyramide (Norpace), and amiodarone (Cordarone)

AFib

Atrial fibrillation (Afib) describes rapid, disorganized atrial beats that are ineffective in emptying the atria so that blood pools and can lead to thrombus formation and emboli. The ventricular rate increases with a decreased stroke volume, and cardiac output decreases with increased myocardial ischemia, resulting in palpitations and fatigue. Afib is caused by coronary artery disease, valvular disease, pulmonary disease, heavy alcohol ingestion, and cardiac surgery. Afib in characterized by a very irregular pulse with an atrial rate of 300–600 bpm and a ventricular rate of 120–200 bpm, and a normal shape and duration (0.4–0.11 seconds) of QRS. Fibrillatory (F) waves are seen instead of P waves. The PR interval cannot be measured, and the P:QRS ratio is highly variable. Afib during sleep is characterized by an irregularly irregular ventricular rhythm and varying rapid oscillations replacing P waves. Treatment may include the following:

- Cardioversion (50–100 joules)
- Ventricular pacing, Amiodarone, propafenone/ibutilide, or electrical cardioversion to convert to sinus rhythm
- β-blockers, diltiazem, amiodarone, or digoxin to control heart rate
- Anticoagulant therapy if Afib persists for more than 24 hours

Prophylaxis

The most common postsurgical arrhythmias are atrial fibrillation (Afib) and atrial flutter (AF). With Afib, the heart rate may be more than 380 bpm but is less than 380 bpm with AF, occurring in up to 30% of patients, even with prophylaxis. Afib and AF occur most often on day 2 or 3 postoperatively.

Prophylaxis reduces the incidence by half. Low-dose β-blockers are administered 12–24 hours after surgery and reduce incidence by 65%:

- Metoprolol, 25–50 mg twice daily, or atenolol, 25 mg daily
- Carvedilol, 3.125–12.5 mg orally twice daily
- Sotalol, 80 mg twice daily
- Dual-site atrial pacing may be used
- Amiodarone may be given by itself or with a β-blocker. Various dosages have been used, including administration of 10 mg/kg daily for 6 preoperative days, continuing postsurgically for a total of 13 days of treatment. Other protocols include administering 200 mg three times daily for 5 preoperative days and 400 mg twice daily for 4–6 postoperative days

Afib postoperative management

Atrial fibrillation (Afib) in the postsurgical patient requires assessment of hemodynamic status and underlying causes as it can decrease cardiac output by 25%–50%. Treatment aims to control rate (of primary concern) and rhythm. Medications used to control rate include β-blockers, calcium channel blockers, and digoxin (although it is less effective than β-blockers). The β-blocker of choice in most cases is metoprolol, while the calcium channel blocker of choice is usually diltiazem. Calcium channel blockers are usually reserved for patients who do not respond to β-blockers. Medications used to convert from Afib include metoprolol, diltiazem, ibutilide, and amiodarone. Ibutilide

is usually used if cardioversion is unsuccessful, but the patient must be monitored carefully for the development of torsade de pointes, a form of ventricular tachycardia in which the QRS complex varies with each heartbeat.

Cardiac arrhythmias

Premature junctional contractions

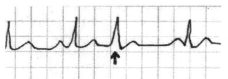 The area around the AV node is the junction, and dysrhythmias that arise from that are called junctional dysrhythmias. Premature junctional contractions (PJCs) occur when a premature impulse starts at the AV node before the next normal sinus impulse reaches the AV node. PJCs are similar to premature atrial contractions (PACs) and generally require no treatment although they may be an indication of digoxin toxicity. The ECG may appear basically normal with an early QRS complex that is normal in shape and duration (0.4 to 0.11 seconds). The P wave may be absent, precede, be part of, or follow the QRS with a PR interval of N0.12 seconds. The P: QRS ratio may vary from <1:1 to 1:1 (with inverted P wave). Rhythm is usually regular at a heart rate of 40 to 60. Significant symptoms related to premature junctional contractions are rare.

Junctional escape beats

Junctional escape beats are delayed heartbeats that occur as a protective mechanism when SA rate of depolarization is slower than the AV node. The junctional escape beats usually arise from the Bundle of His, when atrial impulses are blocked by the AV node. The sinus beat slows intermittently. Junctional beats occur irregularly but may be regular if a junctional escape rhythm develops. Junctional escape rhythms are usually regular with R-R rhythm consistent and a heart rate of 40 to 60 per minute, reflecting the underlying rate of the AV node. Usually P waves are missing or inverted, but this depends on the site the junctional beat originates. When P waves occur, the duration is 0.12 to 0.20 seconds. The QRS segment is < 0.12 seconds.

Junctional rhythms

Junctional rhythms occur when the atrioventricular (AV) node becomes the pacemaker of the heart because the sinus node is depressed from increased vagal tone or block at the AV node, preventing sinus node impulses from being transmitted. While the sinus node normally sends impulses 60–100 bpm, the AV node junction usually sends impulses at 40–60 bpm. The QRS complex is of usual shape and duration (0.4–0.11 seconds). The P wave may be inverted or may be absent, hidden, or after the QRS. If the P wave precedes QRS, the PR interval is less than 0.12 seconds. The P:QRS ratio is less than 1:1 or 1:1. The junctional escape rhythm is a protective mechanism preventing asystole with failure of the sinus node. Slow junctional rhythm is treated with atrial to AV to ventricular pacing and chronotropics.

Accelerated junctional rhythm

Accelerated junctional rhythm is similar to slow junctional rhythm except that with accelerated junctional rhythm the heart rate is 60–100 bpm. Junctional tachycardia, which is rare, occurs with a heart rate of 100–160 bpm. Junctional tachycardia may be paroxysmal, with abrupt starting and stopping, or nonparoxysmal.

Nonparoxysmal AV junctional tachycardia

Nonparoxysmal atrioventricular (AV) junctional tachycardia is characterized by a ventricular rate of 70–100 bpm, is a cardinal sign of digoxin toxicity, but rarely occurs with adequate monitoring of serum levels. It may also be an indication of damage to the AV junction from an acute myocardial infarction.

Nonparoxysmal junctional tachycardia may be chronic. Treatment includes stopping digoxin for those taking it, administering potassium and phenytoin, or beginning digoxin for those not already taking the drug.

AV nodal reentry tachycardia

Atrioventricular (AV) nodal reentry tachycardia occurs when an impulse conducts to area of the AV node, and the impulse is sent in a rapidly repeating cycle back to the same area and to the ventricles, resulting in a fast ventricular rate. The onset and cessation are usually rapid. AV nodal reentry tachycardia (i.e., paroxysmal atrial tachycardia or supraventricular tachycardia if there are no P waves) is characterized by an atrial rate of 150–250 bpm with a ventricular rate of 75–250 bpm, a P wave that is difficult to see or absent, a QRS complex that is usually normal, and a PR interval of less than 0.12 seconds if a P wave is present. The P:QRS ratio is 1–2:1. Precipitating factors include nicotine or caffeine ingestion, hypoxemia, anxiety, and underlying coronary artery disease and cardiomyopathy. Cardiac output may be decreased with a rapid heart rate, causing dyspnea, chest pain, and hypotension. Treatment may include the following:

- Vagal maneuvers (e.g., carotid sinus massage, gag reflex, holding breath)
- Medications (e.g., adenosine, verapamil, diltiazem)
- Cardioversion if other methods unsuccessful

Premature ventricular contractions

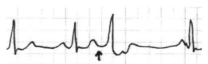

Premature ventricular contractions (PVCs) are those in which the impulse begins in the ventricles and conducts through them before the next sinus impulse. The ectopic QRS complexes may vary in shape, depending on whether there is one (unifocal) or more (multifocal) sites that are stimulating the ectopic beats. PVCs usually cause no morbidity unless there is underlying cardiac disease or an acute myocardial infarction. PVCs are characterized by an irregular heartbeat, a QRS that is 0.12 seconds or more and oddly shaped, a P wave that may be absent or may precede or follow the QRS, a PR interval of less than 0.12 seconds if a P wave is present, and a P:QRS ratio of 0–1:1. Postoperative PVCs may result from alterations in magnesium or potassium levels. Because PVCs may occur with any supraventricular dysrhythmia, the underlying rhythm (e.g., atrial fibrillation) must be noted as well as the PVCs. Treatment includes treating potassium and magnesium alterations, lidocaine, amiodarone, and atrial overdrive pacing.

VT

Ventricular tachycardia (VT) is three or more premature ventricular contractions (PVCs) in a row with a ventricular rate of 100–200 bpm. VT may be triggered by the same things that trigger PVCs and is often related to underlying coronary artery disease, but the rapid rate of contractions make VT dangerous as the ineffective beats may render the person unconscious with no palpable pulse. A detectable rate is usually regular, and the QRS complex is 0.12 seconds or more and is usually abnormally shaped. The P wave may be undetectable with an irregular PR interval if a P wave is present. The P:QRS ratio is often difficult to ascertain because of absence of P waves. Treatment includes defibrillation, amiodarone, and lidocaine.

WCT

Tachycardias are classified as narrow complex or wide complex. Wide and narrow refer to the configuration of the QRS complex wide-complex tachycardia (WCT). About 80% of WCT cases are caused by ventricular tachycardia. WCT originates at some point below the atrioventricular node and may be associated with palpitations, dyspnea, anxiety, and cardiac arrest. Patients may

exhibit diaphoresis. WCT is diagnosed with three or more consecutive beats with a heart rate of over 100 bpm and a QRS duration of 0.12 seconds or more.

NCT

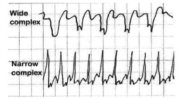

Narrow-complex tachycardia (NCT) is associated with palpitations, dyspnea, and peripheral edema. NCT is generally supraventricular in origin. NCT is diagnosed with three or more consecutive beats with a heart rate of over 100 bpm and a QRS duration of 0.12 seconds or less.

VF

Ventricular fibrillation (VF) is a rapid, very irregular ventricular rate of over 300 bpm with no atrial activity observable on the electrocardiogram (ECG), caused by disorganized electrical activity in the ventricles. The QRS complex is not recognizable as the ECG shows irregular undulations. The causes are the same as for ventricular tachycardia (VT), such as use of alcohol, caffeine, and nicotine or underlying coronary disease, and it may result if VT is not treated. It may also result from an electrical shock or congenital disorder, such as Brugada syndrome. VF is accompanied by lack of a palpable pulse, audible pulse, and respirations and is immediately life-threatening without defibrillation. After emergency defibrillation, the cause should be identified and limited. Mortality is high if VF occurs as part of a myocardial infarction.

Ventricular escape rhythm

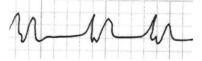

Ventricular escape rhythm

(idioventricular) occurs when the Purkinje fibers below the atrioventricular (AV) node create an impulse. This may occur if the sinus node fails to fire or if there is blockage at the AV node so that the impulse does not go through. Idioventricular rhythm is characterized by a regular ventricular rate of 20–40 bpm. Rates over 40 bpm are called accelerated idioventricular rhythms. The P wave is missing, and the QRS complex has a very bizarre and abnormal shape with a duration of 0.12 seconds or more. The low ventricular rate may cause a decrease in cardiac output, often making the patient lose consciousness. In some patients, the idioventricular rhythm is not associated with low cardiac output.

Ventricular asystole

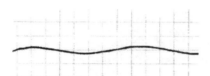

Ventricular asystole is the absence of an audible heartbeat, palpable pulse, and respirations, a condition often referred to as "flat lining" or "cardiac arrest." While the electrocardiogram (ECG) may show some P waves initially, the QRS complex is absent although there may be an occasional QRS "escape beat." Cardiopulmonary resuscitation is required with intubation for ventilation and establishment of an intravenous line for fluids. Without immediate treatment, the patient will suffer from severe hypoxia and brain death within minutes. Identifying the cause is critical for the patient's survival and could include hypoxia, acidosis, electrolyte imbalance, hypothermia, or drug overdose. Even with immediate treatment, the prognosis is poor, and ventricular asystole is often a sign of impending death.

Sinus pause

Sinus pause occurs when the sinus node fails to function properly to stimulate heart contractions and the P wave; there is a pause on the electrocardiogram recording that may persist for a few seconds to a few minutes,

depending on the severity of the dysfunction. A prolonged pause may be difficult to differentiate from cardiac arrest, so the technologist should alert medical personnel if the pause persists more than a few seconds. During the sinus pause, the P wave, QRS complex, and PR and QRS intervals are all absent. The P:QRS ratio is 1:1, and the rhythm is irregular. The pulse rate may vary widely, usually 60–100 bpm. Patients frequently complain of dizziness or syncope.

ECG

The electrocardiogram (ECG) records and shows a graphic display of the electrical activity of the heart through a number of different waveforms, complexes, and intervals:

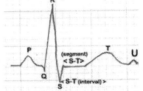

- P wave - The P wave is the start of an electrical impulse in the sinus node that spreads through the atria, initiating muscle depolarization
- QRS complex - The QRS complex represents ventricular muscle depolarization and atrial repolarization
- T wave - The T wave represents ventricular muscle repolarization (resting state) as cells regain negative charge
- U wave - The U wave represents repolarization of the Purkinje fibers.
- A modified 2-lead ECG is often used to monitor basic heart rhythms and dysrhythmias

Typical placement of leads for a 2-lead ECG is 3–5 centimeters inferior to the right clavicle and left lower ribcage. Typical placement for a 3-lead ECG is the right arm near the shoulder, the V_5 position over fifth intercostal space, and the left upper leg near the groin.

12-lead electrocardiogram

The 12-lead electrocardiogram provides a graphic representation of the electrical activity of the heart. It is indicated for chest pain, dyspnea, syncope, acute coronary syndrome, pulmonary embolism, and possible myocardial infarction. It gives a picture of electrical activity from twelve perspectives through the placement of ten body leads:

- Four limb leads are placed distally on the wrists and ankles (but may be placed more proximally if necessary)
- Precordial leads:
  a. V_1: right sternal border at fourth intercostal space
  b. V_2: left sternal border at fourth intercostal space
  c. V_3: midway between V_2 and V_4
  d. V_4: left midclavicular line at fifth intercostal space
  e. V_5: horizontal to V_4 at left anterior axillary line
  f. V_6: horizontal to V_5 at left midaxillary line
- Right-sided leads, which are not always needed, are placed on the right in a mirror image of the left leads, usually to diagnose right ventricular infarction through ST elevation

Heart sounds

Auscultation of heart sounds can help to diagnose different cardiac disorders. Areas to auscultate include the aortic area, pulmonary area, Erb's point, tricuspid area, and the apical area. The normal heart sounds represent closing of the valves.

The first heart sound (S_1), "lub," is closure of the mitral and tricuspid valves (heard at apex/left ventricular area of the heart).

The second heart sound (S_2), "dub," is closure of the aortic and pulmonic valves (heard at the base of the heart). There may be a slight splitting of the S_2.

The time between S_1 and S_2 is systole, and the time between S_2 and the next S_1 is diastole. Systole and diastole should be silent, although ventricular disease can cause gallops, snaps, or clicks, and stenosis of the valves or failure of the valves to close can cause murmurs. Pericarditis may cause a friction rub.

The third heart sound (S3) occurs after the second heart sound (S2) in children and young adults but may indicate heart failure or left ventricular failure in older adults (heard with patient lying on left side).

The fourth heart sound (S4) occurs before the first heart sound (S1) and occurs with ventricular hypertrophy, such as from coronary artery disease, hypertension, or aortic valve stenosis.

Opening snap
Opening snap is an unusual high-pitched sound, occurring after S2 with stenosis of the mitral valve from rheumatic heart disease.

Ejection click
Ejection click is a brief high-pitched sound, occurring immediately after S1 with stenosis of the aortic valve.

Friction rub
Friction rub is a harsh, grating sound heard in systole and diastole with pericarditis.

Murmur
Murmurs are caused by turbulent blood flow from stenotic or malfunctioning valves, congenital defects, or increased blood flow. Murmurs are characterized by location, timing in the cardiac cycle, intensity (rated from grade I to grade VI), pitch (low-to-high pitched), quality (rumbling, whistling, blowing), and radiation to the carotids, axilla, neck, shoulder, or back.

Transvenous pacemakers

Transvenous pacemakers, comprised of a catheter with a lead at the end, may be used prophylactically or therapeutically on a temporary basis to treat a cardiac abnormality, especially bradycardia. The catheter is inserted through a vein at the femoral or neck area and attached to an external pulse generator. Transvenous pacemakers are used to:

- Treat persistent dysrhythmias not responsive to medications
- Increase cardiac output with bradydysrhythmia by increasing rate
- Decrease ventricular or supraventricular tachycardia by "overdrive" stimulation of contractions
- Treat secondary heart block caused by myocardial infarction, ischemia, and drug toxicity
- Improve cardiac output after cardiac surgery
- Provide diagnostic information through electrophysiology studies, which induce dysrhythmias for purposes of evaluation
- Provide pacing when a permanent pacemaker malfunctions

Complications are similar to implanted pacemakers and include increased risk of pacemaker syndrome.

Transcutaneous pacing

Transcutaneous pacing is used temporarily to treat bradydysrhythmia that does not respond to medications (atropine) and results in hemodynamic instability. Generally, an arterial line is placed, and the patient is provided with oxygen before the pacing. The placement of pacing pads (large self-adhesive pads) and electrocardiogram leads varies somewhat, according to the type of equipment, but usually one pacing pad (negative) is placed on the left chest, inferior to the clavicle, and the other (positive) on the left back, inferior to the scapula, so the heart is sandwiched between the two pads so that the myocardium is depolarized through the chest wall. Lead wires attach the pads to the monitor. The rate of pacing is usually set between 60 and 70 bpm. Current is increased slowly until capture occurs—a spiking followed by the QRS sequence—then the current is readjusted downward if possible just to maintain capture. Both demand and fixed modes are available, but the demand mode is preferred. Patients may require analgesia, especially if a higher current setting is needed.

Cardioversion

Cardioversion is a timed electrical stimulation to the heart to convert a tachydysrhythmia (e.g., atrial fibrillation) to a normal sinus rhythm. Usually anticoagulation therapy is administered for at least 3 weeks before elective cardioversion to reduce the risk of emboli, and digoxin is discontinued for at least 48 hours before cardioversion. During the procedure, the patient is usually sedated or anesthetized. Electrodes in the form of gel-covered paddles or pads are positioned in the left chest and left back (in front of and behind the heart), connected by leads to a computerized electrocardiogram (ECG) and cardiac monitor with a defibrillator. The defibrillator is synchronized with the ECG so that the electrical current is delivered during ventricular depolarization (QRS). The timing must be precise to prevent ventricular tachycardia or ventricular fibrillation. Sometimes, drug therapy is used in conjunction with cardioversion; for example, antiarrhythmics (e.g., diltiazem [Cardizem], amiodarone [Cordarone]) may be given before the procedure to slow the heart rate.

Emergency defibrillation

Emergency defibrillation is done to treat acute ventricular fibrillation or ventricular tachycardia in which there is no audible or palpable pulse. A higher voltage is generally used for defibrillation than is used for cardioversion, causing depolarization of myocardial cells, which can then repolarize to regain a normal sinus rhythm. Defibrillation delivers an electrical discharge usually through paddles applied to both sides of the chest. Defibrillation may be repeated, usually up to three times, at increasing voltage, but if the heart has not regained a sinus rhythm by then, cardiopulmonary resuscitation and advanced life support are required. Medications, such as epinephrine or vasopressin may be administered, and cardiopulmonary resuscitation continued for 1 minute, after which defibrillation is again attempted. Additional medications, such as amiodarone, magnesium, or procainamide, may be necessary if there are persistent ventricular dysrhythmias.

Initiating CPB

The patient is heparinized about 3 minutes before initiating cardiopulmonary bypass (CPB) and insertion of cannulas. After the heart is accessed through a midsternal incision/sternotomy, one cannula is placed into the right atrium or femoral vein or dual catheters through the right atrium into the superior and inferior vena cava to provide gravity drainage of venous blood, as the pump system creates a vacuum. (If the aortic valve is incompetent, then the left ventricle must be vented to prevent backflow of blood into the left ventricle.) Note, however, that improper placement of the superior vena cava cannula can result in increased central venous pressure and cerebral edema, and improper placement of the inferior vena cava cannula can cause abdominal vascular distention with inadequate venous return to the CPB machine. A return cannula is usually placed in the ascending aorta but may be placed in the femoral artery. A cross clamp is placed across the aorta (below the return cannula) to divert blood to the CPB machine. (The lungs are not mechanically ventilated during CPB.)

During CPB

During cardiopulmonary bypass (CPB), the blood drains from the cannulas into a venous reservoir and then is pumped through a filter that removes air bubbles or clots. After filtering, a membrane-gas-interface oxygenates the blood to maintain the partial pressure of oxygen with the partial pressure of carbon dioxide at 35–45 mm Hg. The blood goes through a heat exchanger to heat or cool the blood, depending on the stage of the operation. Temperature is usually maintained at 18°C before arrest and 28°C–32°C during surgery and then increased to 37°C before removal from the CPB machine. Cooled blood is more viscous, but it is diluted by crystalloid solutions (commonly 5% dextrose in lactated Ringers). The blood is then pumped back into circulation, bypassing the heart. Cardioplegic potassium-based solution is infused into the aortic root, from which it circulates to the coronary arteries, to ensure cessation of electrical activity, so the heart remains flaccid during CPB; this can result in postoperative hyperkalemia, although excess potassium can be filtered by the CPB machine.

Discontinuation of CPB

To discontinue cardiopulmonary bypass (CPB), the patient must be rewarmed, air evacuated from the system, the aortic cross-clamp opened and removed, and mechanical ventilation restarted. Guidelines for discontinuation include the following:

- Core temperature should be 37°C to prevent metabolic acidosis and decreased myocardial contractility
- Cardiac status must be stable with sinus rhythm (preferable) with evidence of atrioventricular (AV) block. In some cases, increased potassium levels must be treated with calcium, furosemide, or glucose and insulin. AV pacing may be required. Heart rate should be 80–100 bpm. Bradycardia may be treated with pacing or inotropic agents. Cardioversion may be necessary if supraventricular tachycardia occurs. Perfusion should be adequate
- Laboratory values must be checked and within normal limits with a hematocrit of 22%–25%, potassium less than 5.5 mEq/L, and a pH over 7.20
- Monitors must be functioning properly

- Ventilation is resumed with 100% oxygen
- The patient is weaned slowly from CPB. If pump failure occurs as CPB is discontinued, an intra-aortic balloon pump may be used before another attempt to wean the patient

Extracorporeal circulation

Assisted right-heart bypass

Assisted right-heart bypass is sometimes used for off-pump procedures, especially with hypertrophy that interferes with filling of the right ventricle. Devices drain blood from the right atrium and return it to the pulmonary artery.

ECMO

Extracorporeal membrane oxygenation (ECMO) is a modification of the cardiopulmonary bypass equipment that can provide support for the heart and lungs by pumping blood outside of the body for oxygenation. Typically cannula are placed in large vessels, and the blood is pumped to the machine for gas exchange; it is then heated and returned to the arterial system with the venous–arterial type of ECMO or to the venous system with the venous–venous type of ECMO.

Left-heart bypass

Left-heart bypass may be done for thoracic aortic surgery. Blood is drained from the left side of the heart either from the left atrium or inferior pulmonary vein (preferred) with blood returned to the femoral artery or distal aorta (below clamp).

VADs

Ventricular assist devices (VADs) are devices that support circulation with afferent conduits attached to the apex of the left ventricle and an efferent conduit attached to the ascending aorta; each conduit contains a porcine valve that directs flow of blood in one direction. The pump usually rests on the external chest wall and has an attached external pneumatic power source as well as a control circuit.

DHCA

Deep hypothermic circulatory arrest (DHCA) is used primarily for surgery involving the aorta when the aorta cannot be clamped to protect the brain. The patient is cooled to 18°C with the patient's head packed and administration of methylprednisolone (20 mg/g) before clamping the arterial line and draining the blood. Antegrade cerebral perfusion or retrograde cerebral perfusion may also be used.

CPB surgery patients

Medical management

The postoperative care of cardiopulmonary bypass surgery patients requires careful medical management.

Cardiovascular support to maintain adequate cardiac output may require adjustment in heart rate, preload, afterload, and contractility.

Regulation of temperature following hypothermia induced during surgery requires warming but not above 37°C.

Bleeding must be monitored carefully, and autotransfusion devices may be used to replace red blood cells.

Chest tubes must be monitored for patency. "Milking" may cause less tissue damage than "stripping."

Cardiac tamponade may occur if blood accumulates around the heart, requiring surgical intervention.

Respiratory care includes early extubation (usually within 4–8 hours). Supplemental oxygen is given as needed.

Neurological monitoring is necessary for postcardiotomy delirium (e.g., disorientation progressing to agitation, hallucinations, paranoia).

Wound infections may occur, especially if a persistent fever is present. Diabetics may need insulin infusions to maintain glucose levels between 80–110 mg/dL to lower the risk of infection. Hemoglobinuria can result from hemolysis and damage kidney tubules. Urine flow may be increased with furosemide (Lasix) if it is less than 20–30 mL/hr or if it is bloody.

Hypothermia

During cardiopulmonary bypass (CPB), systemic hypothermia (32°C–34°C) is used, but the patient should be warmed to about 36°C before leaving the operating room. Because brain temperature may be higher than measurable core temperature, raising the temperature to 37°C may impair neurocognitive functioning. Peripheral vasoconstriction is often used postoperatively after CPB to provide core warming. Vasodilators redistribute core heat and may slow core warming although they increase perfusion. Heated intravenous fluid and humidifiers in the ventilator circuits may treat hypothermia but are usually not effective for increasing core temperatures. A temperature-controlling system or forced air warming devices, such as the Bair Hugger, may help maintain and increase core temperature. Hypothermia increases the risk of atrial and ventricular arrhythmias. Shivering increases oxygen consumption and the production of carbon dioxide and should be controlled with meperidine.

Hypothermia effects
During the rewarming stage after hypothermia, vasodilation occurs, reducing filling pressures and resulting in hypotension and decreased cardiac output in patients who are hypovolemic. Volume resuscitation must be adequate to maintain filling pressures, especially in the first 6 postoperative hours, but overloading the patient with fluid (> 2 L every 6 hours) may result in hemodilution, requiring blood transfusions and plasma or platelets to increase clotting factors and prevent bleeding. Generally, fluids should be limited to 1500–1750 mL/24 hr or no more than 20 mL/kg. The usual initial bolus of fluid is 500 mL of lactated Ringers or normal saline. Colloids should be avoided with capillary leak syndrome but are indicated for hypotension primarily related to peripheral vasodilation. With marginal hypotension, fluids are provided to increase pulmonary artery diastolic pressure or pulmonary capillary wedge pressure to 18–20 mm Hg first with crystalloid and then colloid. If a patient remains hypotensive and the cardiac index (CI) is less than 2.2 L/min/m², pure α phenylephrine is provided. With a CI of 1.8–2.2 L/min/m², an α and β norepinephrine is provided. If the CI falls to less than 1.8 L/min/m², an inotrope and norepinephrine are provided as needed.

Dealing with hypothermia effects
Hypothermic vasoconstriction occurs with core temperatures less than 35°C–36°C, increasing systemic vascular resistance (SVR) and resulting in hypertension. Treatment includes inotropes for a cardiac index less than 2 L/min/m² in conjunction with fluid replacement until systolic pressure is 100–120 mm Hg and pulmonary artery diastolic pressure or pulmonary capillary wedge pressure is 15–20 mm Hg. Warming methods should be used to increase core temperature to 36°C. Vasodilators used to treat hypothermic vasoconstriction include nicardipine and clevidipine. Vasodilators reduce afterload, restore preload to adequate levels, and improve peripheral perfusion, reducing SVR and blood pressure. Preload should be maintained 20 mm Hg or less but prevented from falling too low as this may precipitate hypovolemia and hypotension. If the cardiac index falls below 2 L/min/m² with adequate filling pressures but mild hypertension in a patient receiving an

inotropic agent, a low-dose vasodilator may be provided. Care should be used when discontinuing an inotropic agent unless cardiac output is adequate because vasoconstriction may be a compensatory mechanism to maintain cardiac function.

Diuresis/hypotension

Diuresis in the cardiac postoperative period may result in the production of copious quantities of urine, causing lowered filling pressures, decreased cardiac output, and hypotension. Cardiopulmonary bypass often results in relative diuresis of 200–400 mL/hr because of hemodilution and drugs that affect osmosis, so urinary output is not a good indication of perfusion in the first few hours after surgery. Identifying the cause of diuresis is important to provide compensatory treatment when needed. Causes may include:

- Vasoactive drugs, such as nesiritide, fenoldopam, or dopamine (provided during surgery to promote renal function). It may be necessary to change medications to low-dose epinephrine, milrinone, or dobutamine
- Furosemide, which is provided during surgery; increased fluids may be required
- Mannitol, which is provided during surgery; increased fluids may be required
- Hyperglycemia (blood glucose maintained at less than 180 mg/dL)

A response to hemodilution and increased interstitial fluid or crystalloid and colloid administration; care must be taken to avoid excess colloid, which can produce hemodilution.

Pathophysiologic changes

Cardiopulmonary bypass (CPB) is associated with a number of pathophysiologic changes that must be monitored and evaluated:
- Decreased concentration of plasma proteins from hemodilution and absorption onto bypass circuit's increased inflammatory response and capillary permeability
- Increased epinephrine, norepinephrine for 24 hours after surgery, increasing systemic resistance; increased cortisol level for 24 hours, increasing sodium retention and potassium excretion
- Hyperglycemia from hormonal stress
- Decreased level of triiodothyronine
- Pulmonary dysfunction (decreases surfactant effects, compliance, and functional residual volume, increasing shunts)
- Progressive hypothermia (after drop) from chest remaining open after CPB
- Coagulopathy because of disruption of the coagulation system, hemodilution from crystalloids that reduce platelets and clotting factors, and activation of platelets in contact with the extracorporeal circuit
- Activation of renin–aldosterone system, increasing sodium retention and potassium excretion; elevation of angiotensin II levels, increasing sodium retention and renal vasoconstriction
- Release of vasoactive substances: nitric oxide ns prostacyclin, which impairs reabsorption of solutes, and complement, kallikrein, and bradykinin, which increase an inflammatory response

Decreased SVR management

Decreased systemic vascular resistance (SVR), also referred to as vasodilatory shock, occurs in 5%–8% of patients after cardiac surgery with cardiopulmonary bypass (CPB) with normal or increased cardiac output, perhaps associated with an inflammatory response to CPB. Patients exhibit an abrupt and precipitous fall in arterial blood pressure with tachycardia as a response to decreased SVR. Hypoperfusion can lead to vasodilation, which, in turn, can lead to systemic inflammatory response syndrome and multiorgan dysfunction syndrome. Patients with an ejection fraction of less than 35% are at increased risk as are those requiring ventricular assist devices. Initial treatment includes fluid resuscitation, reduction in afterload, inotropes to increase contractility, and norepinephrine to increase blood pressure through vasoconstriction. If this is ineffective, vasopressin may be administered or methylene blue, if vasopressin is ineffective.

Removal of lines and tubes

Swan-Ganz catheter
When the patient is stabilized to the point of not needing inotropes and vasodilators, the Swan-Ganz catheter is removed.

Central lines
Central lines are removed when they are no longer needed for monitoring.

Arterial lines
Arterial lines are removed after extubation and a stable arterial blood gas (ABG). A subsequent ABG after a period on room air must also be obtained. Lines should not be maintained solely for blood sampling.

Left atrial line
The left atrial line is removed before chest tubes are removed in case intrapericardial bleeding occurs when the line is removed.

Chest tubes
Chest tubes are removed when drainage is less than 100 mL/8 hr. Suction should be turned off before removal of mediastinal tubes. Chest x-ray is done after removal of pleural chest tubes to evaluate for pneumothorax.

Pleural drain
A pleural drain (lateral chest wall) is removed 3–5 days after surgery.

Urinary catheter
When the patient is no longer receiving pronounced diuresis, does not have a risk of urinary retention, and is mobile (usually at the beginning of day 2), the urinary catheter is removed.

Heart transplantation

Heart transplantation is similar to other open-heart procedures in that cardiopulmonary bypass is needed during the procedure. The sternotomy and thymectomy are performed and then the pericardial sac is opened to expose the heart. If the donor heart is larger than the recipient's, the left pericardium, sparing the phrenic nerve, may be removed. In orthotopic transplantation, the most commonly used, the posterior portion of the left atrium is left for attachment of the new heart, but the rest of the heart is excised. The donor heart is trimmed and sutured to fit with the remnants of the old heart. If there are a number of structural anomalies, such as transposition of the great vessels, then reconstruction of vessels may be needed during the procedure. Once the new heart is in place, the heart is taken off bypass and is stimulated to begin contractions. In heterotopic transplantation (rare), the new heart is sutured to the old heart, joining the chambers and creating a "double" heart.

Heart transplant patients

Postoperative management of heart transplant patients is similar to that of other cardiac surgeries. Treatments include the following:
- Mechanical ventilation is used initially, but respiratory care with adequate ventilation must be monitored constantly, especially if the donor heart was larger than the native heart, resulting in compression of the lungs
- Intravenous fluids and various medications, such as sedation and vasodilators, are administered
- Antithymocyte globulin, azathioprine, cyclosporine or tacrolimus may be used for immunosuppression as well as corticosteroids (methylprednisolone).

- 18 -

Intravenous immunosuppressive drugs are given after surgery, but these are switched to oral medications as soon as possible. Protocols are established at each institution and may vary. Medication doses are age dependent

The risk for rejection is the greatest in the first few months and close follow-up is necessary with routine laboratory tests, including echocardiograms, chest x-rays, and blood tests.

Amylase and pancreatitis level increase

A transient period of increased amylase levels (hyperamylasemia) occurs in up to 65% of patients after cardiopulmonary bypass (CPB), but only 3% or less develop pancreatitis. Transient hyperamylasemia can occur with both on-pump and off-pump procedures and may result from decreased excretion through the kidneys. If levels are elevated to 1000 IU/L or more in the early postoperative period, the risk of developing pancreatitis, increases so patients need careful observation. Indications include nausea, lack of appetite, and ileus. Treatment is supportive. Pancreatitis usually results from ischemia that causes necrosis, often associated with prolonged CPB and persistent low-cardiac output. Patients with a history of alcoholism are at increased risk. Pancreatitis may cause fever, elevated white blood cell count, abdominal distention, abdominal pain, nausea, vomiting, and paralytic ileus. Pancreatitis may be present without marked increase in amylase levels. Treatment includes insertion of a nasogastric tube and antibiotics. Surgical debridement may be necessary in severe cases.

Pulse oximetry

Pulse oximetry, continuous or intermittent, uses an external oximeter that attaches to the patient's finger or earlobe to measure arterial oxygen saturation (SpO_2), the percentage of hemoglobin that is saturated with oxygen. The oximeter also usually attaches to a machine that emits a beep with each heartbeat and indicates the current heart rate. Blood pressure monitoring is also necessary. The oximeter uses light waves to determine SpO_2. In patients with pronounced vasoconstriction, the earlobe may provide more accurate readings than the finger. It is important to maintain SpO_2 at 95% or more, although some patients with chronic respiratory disorders, such as chronic obstructive pulmonary disease may have a low SpO_2. If SpO_2 falls, the oximeter should be repositioned, as incorrect position is a common cause of inaccurate readings. Oximetry is often used postoperatively to assess peripheral circulation and when patients are on mechanical ventilation. Oximeters do not provide information about carbon dioxide levels, so they cannot monitor carbon dioxide retention. Oximeters cannot differentiate between different forms of hemoglobin, so if hemoglobin has picked up carbon dioxide, the oximeter will not recognize that.

Jugular venous pressure

Jugular venous pressure (neck vein) is used to assess the cardiac output and pressure in the right heart as the pulsations relate to changes in pressure in the right atrium. This procedure is usually not accurate if the pulse rate is 100 bpm or more. This is a noninvasive estimation of central venous pressure and waveform. Measurement should be done with the internal jugular if possible; if not, the external jugular may be used. Elevate the patient's head to 45° (and to 90° if necessary) with the patient's head turned to the opposite side of the examination.

Position a light at an angle to illuminate veins and shadows.

Measure the height of the jugular vein pulsation above the sternal joint, using a ruler.

Normal height is 4 cm or less above the sternal angle.

Increased pressure (> 4 cm) indicates increased pressure in the right atrium and right heart failure. It may also indicate pericarditis or tricuspid stenosis. Laughing or coughing may trigger or increase the Valsalva response.

Compartment syndrome

Compartment syndrome occurs when the myofascial compartment size decreases because of constriction or contents of a compartment increase (usually swelling, hemorrhage, or infiltrated intravenous line). However, prolonged cardiopulmonary bypass (CPB) may result in ischemic/reperfusion injury to a lower extremity, especially if retrograde reperfusion is in the femoral artery. The increased compartment pressure reduces capillary perfusion below the level necessary for tissue viability and damages nerves:

- Normal values: 0–8 mm Hg
- Compartment syndrome: 30–40 mm Hg or higher

Edema of the involved lower extremity is common after surgery, but if ischemia persists for 4–6 hours, then pressures should be measured. Symptoms include the "six Ps": paresthesia, pain (i.e., deep, throbbing, relentless pain and positive Homan's sign for lower extremities), pressure, pallor, paralysis, and pulselessness in the peripheral pulses (although this may indicate arterial occlusion rather than compartment syndrome). Surgical fasciotomy may be necessary if elevation of the limb is not effective in reducing pressure.

Cardiac surgery complications

Cardiac tamponade

Cardiac tamponade occurs with pericardial effusion, causing pressure against the heart. It may be a complication of trauma, pericarditis, cardiac surgery, or heart failure. About 50 mL of fluid normally circulates in the pericardial area to reduce friction, and a sudden increase in this volume can compress the heart, causing a number of cardiac responses:

- Increased end-diastolic pressure in both ventricles
- Decrease in venous return
- Decrease in ventricular filling

Symptoms may include pressure or pain in the chest, dyspnea, and pulsus paradoxus of 10 mm Hg or more. Beck's triad (i.e., increased central venous pressure, causing distended neck veins; a fall in arterial pressure; distant muffled heart sounds) is common. A sudden decrease in chest tube drainage can occur as fluid and clots accumulate in the pericardial sac, preventing the blood from filling the ventricles and decreasing cardiac output and perfusion of the body, including the kidneys (resulting in decreased urinary output). X-rays may show a change in cardiac silhouette and mediastinal shift (in 20%). Treatment includes pericardiocentesis with a large bore needle or surgical repair to control bleeding and relieve cardiac compression.

Pericardiocentesis

Pericardiocentesis is done with ultrasound guidance to diagnose pericardial effusion or with an electrocardiogram (ECG) or ultrasound guidance to relieve cardiac tamponade. Pericardiocentesis may be done as treatment for cardiac arrest or with presentation of pulseless electrical activity with increased jugular venous pressure. Nonhemorrhagic tamponade may be relieved in 60%–90% of cases, but hemorrhagic tamponade requires thoracotomy, as blood will continue to accumulate until the cause of hemorrhage is corrected. Resuscitation equipment must be available, including a defibrillator; an intravenous line must be in place; and cardiac monitoring must be instituted:

- The chest is elevated to 45° to bring the heart closer to chest wall
- Premedication with atropine may prevent vasovagal reactions
- If abdominal distention is present, a nasogastric tube should be inserted
- After insertion of the needle, the obturator is removed, and a syringe is attached for aspiration. A sterile alligator clamp is attached from the needle to any precordial lead of the ECG for monitoring to ensure that the ventricle is not punctured
- Postprocedure chest x-ray should be done to check for a pneumothorax

Upper GI bleeding

Upper gastrointestinal (GI) bleeding can occur with both on-pump and off-pump cardiac surgeries, usually from development of a duodenal stress ulceration because of ischemia and hypoperfusion/reperfusion injury. Mortality rates associated with upper GI bleeding are 15%–20%. Risk factors include a history of gastric disorders (i.e., gastritis, ulcers) and advanced age. Postoperative conditions that increase risk include decreased cardiac output, coagulopathy, anticoagulation, and prolonged mechanical ventilation. Indications include bright red drainage from a nasogastric (NG) tube, vomiting of blood, or bloody stools. Preventive measures include sucralfate, 1 g every 6 hours (orally [po] or per NG tube) or proton pump inhibitors (pantoprazole, 40 mg intravenously or po; omeprazole, 20 mg daily po; lansoprazole, 15 mg daily po; rabeprazole, 10 mg daily po). Those receiving acetylsalicylic acid should receive enteric-coated preparations. Treatment includes upper GI endoscopy with laser bipolar coagulation and somatostatin, 250 μg/hr for 5 days, for severe bleeding.

Lower GI bleeding

Lower gastrointestinal (GI) bleeding can occur with mesenteric ischemia, ischemic colitis associated with extended hypoperfusion, Clostridium difficile or other super infection from antibiotics, anticoagulation (i.e., bleeding polyps, lesions), and intestinal angiodysplasia (i.e., Heyde's syndrome, which can occur with aortic stenosis). Indications include melena, blood-streaked stool, or frank rectal bleeding. Upper GI bleeding is ruled out with insertion of a nasogastric tube, followed by sigmoidoscopy or colonoscopy to identify the cause and site of bleeding. Underlying coagulopathy or other cause must be identified and treated. Treatment may include mesenteric angiography and vasopressin infusion; embolotherapy; octreotide, 50 μg over 50 minutes; or somatostatin, 50 μg bolus with follow-up infusion of 250 μg/hr. On rare occasions, surgical intervention may be necessary.

RBC tests

Total RBCs
Total RBCs:
- Males over 18 years: 4.5–5.5 million/mm3
- Females over 18 years: 4.0–5.0 million/mm3

Hemoglobin
Hemoglobin carries oxygen and is decreased in anemia and increased in polycythemia. Normal values:
- Males over 18 years: 14.0–17.46 g/dL
- Females over 18 years: 12.0–16.0 g/dL

Hematocrit
Hematocrit indicates the proportion of RBCs in a liter of blood (usually about three times the hemoglobin number). Normal values:
- Males over 18 years: 45%–52%.
- Females over 18 years: 36%–¬48%

MCV
Mean corpuscular volume (MCV) indicates the size of RBCs and can differentiate types of anemia. For adults, a MCV of less than 80 μm3

is microcytic and over 100 μm3 is macrocytic. Normal values:

- Males over 18 years: 84–96 μm3
- Females over 18 years: 76–96 μm3

MCHC

Mean corpuscular hemoglobin concentration (MCHC) indicates the average concentration of hemoglobin in each cell (Hb/RBC = MCHC). Normal values:

- Males and females over 18 years: 30–35 g/dL and 30%–35%

Reticulocyte count

Reticulocyte count measures marrow production and should rise with anemia. Normal values: 0.5%–1.5% of total RBCs

DIC

Disseminated intravascular coagulation (DIC), also known as consumption coagulopathy, is a secondary disorder that is triggered by another, such as trauma, congenital heart disease, necrotizing enterocolitis, sepsis, and severe viral infections. DIC triggers both coagulation and hemorrhage through a complex series of events that includes trauma that causes tissue factor (transmembrane glycoprotein) to enter the circulation and bind with coagulation factors, triggering the coagulation cascade. This stimulates thrombin to convert fibrinogen to fibrin, causing aggregation and destruction of platelets and forming clots that can be disseminated throughout the intravascular system. These clots increase in size as platelets adhere to the clots, causing blockage of both the microvascular systems and larger vessels, and this can result in ischemia and necrosis. Clot formation triggers fibrinolysis and plasmin to breakdown fibrin and fibrinogen, causing destruction of clotting factors, resulting in hemorrhage. Both processes, clotting and hemorrhage, continue at the same time, placing the patient at high risk for death, even with treatment.

Symtoms and treatment

The onset of symptoms of disseminated intravascular coagulation (DIC) may be very rapid or progress slowly, resulting in a chronic form of the disease. Those who develop chronic disease usually have fewer acute symptoms and may slowly develop ecchymosis or bleeding wounds.

Signs and Symptoms	Treatment
Bleeding from surgical or venous puncture sites Evidence of gastrointestinal bleeding with distention and bloody diarrhea Hypotension and acute symptoms of shock Petechiae and purpura with extensive bleeding into the tissues Laboratory abnormalities: Prolonged prothrombin and partial thromboplastin times Decreased platelet counts and fragmented red blood cells Decreased fibrinogen	Identifying and treating underlying cause Replacement blood products, such as platelets and fresh frozen plasma Anticoagulation therapy (heparin) to increase clotting time Cryoprecipitate to increase fibrinogen levels Coagulation inhibitors and coagulation factors

Coagulation profile

The coagulation profile measures clotting mechanisms, identifies clotting disorders, screens preoperative patients, and diagnoses excessive bruising and bleeding. Values vary depending on the laboratory.

Postoperative complications: Coagulation profile

Prothrombin time (PT)	10–14 seconds	PT increases with anticoagulation therapy, vitamin K deficiency, decreased prothrombin, disseminated intravascular coagulation (DIC), liver disease, and malignant neoplasm. Some drugs many shorten time.
Partial thromboplastin time (PTT)	30–45 seconds	PTT increases with hemophilia A and B, von Willebrand's, vitamin deficiency, lupus, DIC, and liver disease.
Activated partial thromboplastin time (aPTT)	21–35 seconds	This is similar to PTT but decreases in extensive cancer, early DIC, and after acute hemorrhage; aPTT is used to monitor heparin dosage.
Thrombin clotting time (TCT) or thrombin time (TT)	7–12 seconds (< 21)	TT is used most often to determine the dosage of heparin; prolonged with multiple myeloma, abnormal fibrinogen, uremia, and liver disease.
Bleeding time	2–9.5 minutes	Using the Ivy method on the forearm, bleeding time increases with DIC, leukemia, renal failure, aplastic anemia, von Willebrand's, some drugs, and alcohol.
Platelet count	150– 400,000/mm³	There will be increased bleeding with fewer than 50,000/mm³ platelets and increased clotting with more than 750,000/mm³.

DIC panel

Disseminated intravascular coagulation (DIC) panel includes a number of tests. Generally, test results that measure materials needed for clotting are decreased and those that measure clotting times are increased. Typical findings that indicate DIC include the following:

Activated partial thromboplastin time (aPTT)	Increased time
Prothrombin time	Findings vary, including increased time (in 75%), normal time (in 25%), or shortened time (in 25%)
Partial thromboplastin time	Increased time (in 50%–60%)
Thrombin time	Increased
D-dimer	D-dimer, a specific polymer that results when fibrin breaks down, giving a marker to indicate the degree of fibrinolysis, increased (usually more reliable than FSP)
Fibrinogen	Decreased
Platelets	Less than 100,000/mm³
Fibrin split products (FSP)	Increased (in 75%–100%). FSPs occur as more clots form and more breakdown of fibrinogen and fibrin occur, interfering with blood coagulation by coating platelets, disrupting thrombin, and attaching to fibrinogen so stable clots cannot form.
Clotting factor assays (V, VI, VII, X, XIII)	Decreased
Antithrombin III	Decreased (in 90%)

NSTEMI

Non–ST-segment elevation myocardial infarction (NSTEMI) ST elevation on the electrocardiogram (ECG) occurs in response to myocardial damage resulting from infarction or severe ischemia. The absence of ST elevation may be diagnosed as unstable angina or NSTEMI, but cardiac enzyme levels increase with NSTEMI, indicating partial blockage of coronary arteries with some damage. Symptoms are consistent with unstable angina, with chest pain or tightness, pain radiating to the neck or arm, dyspnea, anxiety, weakness, dizziness, nausea, vomiting, and "heartburn." Initial treatment may include nitroglycerin, β-blockers, antiplatelet agents, or antithrombotic agents. Ongoing treatment may include β-blockers, aspirin, statins, angiotensin-converting enzyme inhibitors, angiotensin-receptor blockers, and clopidogrel. Percutaneous coronary intervention is not recommended.

STEMI

This more severe type of MI involves complete blockage of one or more coronary arteries with myocardial damage, resulting in ST elevation. Symptoms are those of acute MI. As necrosis occurs, Q waves often develop, indicating irreversible myocardial damage, which may result in death, so treatment involves immediate reperfusion before necrosis can occur.

MIs

Myocardial infarctions (MIs) are classified according to their location and the extent of injury. Transmural MI involves the full thickness of the heart (i.e., the endocardium, myocardium, epicardium), often producing a series of Q waves on the electrocardiogram (ECG). An MI most frequently damages the left ventricle and the septum, but the right ventricle may be damaged, depending upon the damaged area:

- Anterior wall infarction occurs with occlusion in the proximal left anterior descending artery and may damage the left ventricle
- Left lateral wall infarction occurs with occlusion of the circumflex coronary artery, often causing damage to anterior wall as well
- Inferior wall infarction occurs with occlusion of the right coronary artery and causes conduction malfunctions
- Right ventricular infarction occurs with occlusion of the proximal section of the right coronary artery and damages the right ventricle and the inferior wall
- Posterior wall infarction occurs with occlusion in the right coronary artery or circumflex artery and may be difficult to diagnose

Acute coronary syndromes

Myocardial infarctions (MIs), formerly classified as transmural or nontransmural, are currently classified as Q-wave or non–Q-wave or ST-segment elevation MI (STEMI) or non–ST-segment elevation MI (NSTEMI).

Q-wave and non–Q-wave myocardial infarctions

Q-wave (STEMI)	Non–Q-wave (NSTEMI)
Q-wave MI is characterized by a series of abnormal Q waves (wider and deeper) on electrocardiogram (ECG), especially in the early morning, related to adrenergic activity and ST-segment elevation. Infarction is usually prolonged and results in necrosis. Coronary occlusion is complete in 80%–90%. Q-wave MI is often, but not always, transmural. Peak creatine kinase (CK) levels occur in about 27 hours. Mortality rates are about 10%.	Non–Q-wave MI is characterized by changes in the ST-T wave with ST depression (usually reversible). Usually reperfusion occurs spontaneously, so infarct size is smaller. Contraction necrosis related to reperfusion is common. Non–Q-wave MI is usually nontransmural. Coronary occlusion is complete in only 20%–30%. Peak CK levels occur in 12–13 hours. Mortality rates are about 2–3%. Reinfarction is common, so 2-year survival rates are similar to Q-wave MI.

Clinical manifestations of MI

Clinical manifestations of myocardial infarction (MI) may vary considerably, with men presenting with the "classic" symptom of sudden onset of crushing chest pain and women and those under 55 presenting with atypical symptoms. Diabetic patients may have a reduced sensation of pain because of neuropathy and may complain primarily of weakness. Elderly patients may also have neuropathic changes that reduce the sensation of pain. More than half of all patients present with acute MIs with no prior symptoms of cardiovascular disease. Symptoms may include the following:

- Angina with chest pain that may radiate to neck or arms
- Palpitations
- Hypertension or hypotension
- Changes on the electrocardiogram, such as ST-segment and T-wave changes, tachycardia, bradycardia, and dysrhythmias
- Dyspnea
- Pulmonary edema and dependent edema
- Nausea and vomiting
- Decreased urinary output
- Pallor, cold and clammy skin, and diaphoresis
- Neurological or psychological disturbances, such as anxiety, light-headedness, headache, visual abnormalities, slurred speech, and fear

Papillary muscle rupture

The atrioventricular valves separate the atria from the ventricles with the tricuspid valve on the right and the bicuspid (mitral) valve on the left. The papillary muscles are located on the sides of ventricular walls and connect to the valves with fibrous bands called chordae tendineae. During systole, the papillary muscles contract, tightening the chordae tendineae and closing the valves. One complication of a myocardial infarction (MI) is papillary muscle rupture, usually on the left, affecting the mitral valve, with the posteromedial papillary muscle more often affected than the anterolateral. Dysfunction of the papillary muscles occurs in about 40% of those with a posterior septal infarction, but rupture can occur with infarction of the inferior wall or an anterolateral MI. Rupture on the right side results in tricuspid regurgitation and right ventricular failure while rupture on the left side leads to mitral regurgitation with resultant pulmonary edema and cardiogenic shock. Early identification and surgical repair are critical.

Cardiogenic shock

Cardiogenic shock in adults most often is secondary to myocardial infarction damage that reduces the contractility of the ventricles, interfering with the pumping mechanism of the heart and decreasing oxygen perfusion. Cardiogenic shock may occur as a postoperative complication. Cardiogenic shock has three characteristics: increased preload, increased afterload, and decreased contractility. Together these result in decreased cardiac output and an increase in systemic vascular resistance to compensate and protect vital organs. This results in an increase of afterload in the left ventricle with an increased need for oxygen. As the cardiac output continues to decrease, tissue perfusion decreases, coronary artery perfusion decreases, fluid backs up, and the left ventricle fails to pump the blood adequately, resulting in pulmonary edema and right ventricular failure.

Symptoms	Treatment
Hypotension with systolic blood pressure less than 90 mm Hg Tachycardia over 100 bpm with a weak thready pulse and dysrhythmias Decreased heart sounds Chest pain Tachypnea and basilar rales Cool, moist skin, and pallor	Intravenous fluids Inotropic agents Antidysrhythmics Intra-aortic balloon pump or left ventricular assist device

DVT

Deep vein thrombosis (DVT) is usually related to poor circulation or damage to vessels and is more common in patients over 40 years of age. DVT is associated with inactivity (e.g., during flying) and surgery and should be differentiated from other injuries when patients complain of calf pain. Homan's sign (i.e., pain in the palpated calf on dorsiflexion of the ankle) occurs in only 10%.

Signs and Symptoms	Treatment
No overt symptoms (in some) Unilateral leg edema Pain and tenderness Erythema Temperature over 38°C (100.4°F) Edema and cyanosis of the lower extremities (with involvement of the inferior vena cava) Increased risk of embolization, including pulmonary embolism	Bed rest with elevation of extremity above the heart Warm compresses Elastic compression stockings (Class II: 30–40 mm Hg) when able to ambulate (used for 3–6 months) Anticoagulants (e.g., unfractionated heparin, low-molecular-weight heparins, hirudin derivatives, warfarin) Surgical intervention (e.g., venous thrombectomy, insertion of vena cava interruption devices) Analgesia

Acute VTE

Acute venous thromboembolism (VTE) is a condition that includes both deep vein thrombosis (DVT) and pulmonary emboli (PE). VTE may be precipitated by invasive procedures, lack of mobility, and inflammation, so it is a common complication in critical care units. Virchow's triad comprises common risk factors:

- blood stasis
- injury to endothelium
- hypercoagulability

Some patients may be initially asymptomatic, but symptoms may include the following:
- Aching or throbbing pain

- Positive Homan's sign (pain in calf when foot is dorsiflexed)
- Erythema and edema
- Dilation of vessels
- Cyanosis

Diagnosis may be made by ultrasound or the D-dimer test, which tests the serum for cross-linked fibrin derivatives. Computed tomography scan, pulmonary angiogram, and a ventilation–perfusion lung scan may be used to diagnose pulmonary emboli. Prophylaxis is very important, but once diagnosed, treatment involves bed rest, elevation of the affected limb, anticoagulation therapy, and analgesics. Elastic stockings are worn when the patient begins ambulating.

Edema

Edema is an indication of hypervolemia-associated hyponatremia, so cardiac surgical patients should be monitored for peripheral and depending edema. Edema is usually checked by pressing the index finger into the tissue on top of each foot, behind the medial malleolus, and over the shin, starting distally and moving proximally to the highest level of edema, comparing both legs:
Edema is rated on a 1–4 point scale:
- 1+ slight pitting to about 2 mm (persists 10–15 seconds)
- 2+ moderate pitting to about 4 mm (persists 10–15 seconds)
- 3+ moderately severe pitting to about 6 mm (persists > 1 minute)
- 4+ severe pitting to 8 mm or more (persists 2–5 minutes)

Venous edema is edema from the ankle to the knee and may involve some limitation in ankle movement. Dependent pitting edema occurs but may become nonpitting in chronic disease.

Lymphedema is usually unilateral nonpitting hard edema from the toes to the groin. Lipedema is symmetrical bilateral soft rubbery tissue from the ankle to the groin and sometimes hips with pain on palpation and frequent bruising.

Thrombocytopenia

Thrombocytopenia occurs when the platelet count drops to less than 50,000/mm³, putting the patient at high risk for bleeding from trauma injury or conditions that affect blood coagulation (i.e., hemophilia, liver disease). Thrombocytopenia may occur with cardiac surgery because of hemodilution or destruction of platelets during extracorporeal circulation or from intra-aortic balloon pump (IABP). Platelet counts usually improve within a few days. Other causes include some medications (i.e., heparin, inamrinone) and sepsis. After surgery, thrombocytopenia may manifest as impaired hemostasis. When the platelet count drops below 20,000/mm³, the patient may have spontaneous bleeding. Treatment includes platelet transfusions for counts less than 20,000–30,000/mm³. If persistent bleeding occurs, transfusions are given if the count is less than 100,000/mm³, although, with platelet dysfunction, transfusions may be administered at higher counts. If the patient is to undergo a planned surgical procedure, such as IABP removal, then transfusions are given at 60,000/mm³ or less to reduce the risk of intraoperative and postoperative bleeding.

HIT and HITTS

Heparin-induced thrombocytopenia (HIT) and thrombosis syndrome (HITTS) occur in patients receiving heparin for anticoagulation.

Type I
Type I is a transient condition, occurring within a few days and causing depletion of platelets (< 100,000/mm³), but heparin may be continued as the condition usually resolves without intervention.

Type II
Type II is an autoimmune reaction to heparin that occurs in 3%–5% of those receiving

unfractionated heparin and also occurs with low-molecular-weight heparin. It is characterized by low platelets (< 150,000/mm^3) that are 50% or more below baseline. Onset is after 5–14 days, but it can occur within hours of reheparinization. Death rates are 30% or fewer. Heparin-antibody complexes form and release platelet factor 4 (PF4), which attracts heparin molecules and adheres to platelets and endothelial lining, stimulating thrombin and platelet clumping. This puts the patient at risk for thrombosis and vessel occlusion rather than hemorrhage, causing stroke, myocardial infarction, and limb ischemia with symptoms associated with the site of thrombosis. Treatment includes discontinuation of all heparin products and administration of direct thrombin inhibitors (e.g., lepirudin, argatroban).

Alternative to heparin

Argatroban	Direct thrombin inhibitor	Indicated as treatment for those with heparin-induced thrombocytopenia (HIT) or at risk for HIT undergoing percutaneous coronary intervention (PCI) Metabolized through the liver so used for those with renal impairment but affects INR so transition to warfarin must be done carefully Starting dose: 2 µg/kg/min after effects of heparin have subsided Maintenance dose: 0.5 to 1.2 µg/kg/min Monitored: Partial thromboplastin time (PTT) with a goal of 1.5–3 times baseline
Desirudin	Direct thrombin inhibitor	Used for prevention of deep venous thrombosis (DVT), for patients at risk for heparin-induced thrombocytopenia (HIT), and for thrombosis prophylaxis for cardiac surgery; does not lead to formation of heparin antibodies Effect on INR is less than with argatroban Dosage: 15 mg subcutaneously twice a day; reduced dosage given for renal impairment Monitored: partial thromboplastin time (PTT) and signs of bleeding
Lepirudin	Direct thrombin inhibitor	Usually drug of choice for those at risk for HIT Starting dose: 0.2–0.4 mg/kg bolus Maintenance dose: infusion of 0.2 mg/hg/hr (continuous) Monitored: PTT with a goal of 1.5–2.5 times baseline
abigatran	Direct thrombin inhibitor	Used to prevent strokes with atrial fibrillation; reduced risk of stroke compared to warfarin but increased risk of gastrointestinal bleeding Withheld during invasive or surgical procedures and then restarted Dosage: 150 mg orally twice daily; 75 mg given with renal impairment Monitor: activated PTT; PTT and INR are insensitive to drug, thrombin time for direct thrombin inhibitors, or ecarin clotting time

Reversal of anticoagulation

Protamine

Protamine is used to reverse anticoagulation caused by a heparin overdose. It is administered slowly intravenously over 10 minutes and binds with heparin, eliminating its anticoagulant properties. Doses should not exceed 50 mg. It should be given undiluted but may be administered in 5% dextrose in water or normal saline. It should not be given with other drugs, as it is incompatible with some antibiotics. Each unit of protamine neutralizes about 100 USP U of heparin.

Vitamin K

Vitamin K (phytonadione [AcquaMEPHYTON]), preferably in oral form, is used to reverse anticoagulation caused by an overdose of warfarin (Coumadin) or superwarfarin (Ramik), found in rodenticides. Drug interactions can increase or decrease prothrombin times. Vitamin K requires hours to work, so packed red blood cells or fresh frozen plasma may be needed in emergency situations. Vitamin K is given only if prothrombin times are elevated, not prophylactically. Doses vary with the amount of ingestion and are given three to four times daily, usually 2–20 mg initially for warfarin and 50–150 mg for superwarfarin. Superwarfarin ingestion may require treatment for over 8 weeks.

Controling postoperative bleeding

Recombinant activated factor VII
This drug activates the extrinsic pathway of coagulation and stimulates production of thrombin, platelet activation, and the formation of fibrin clots, improving prothrombin time. While indicated for those with clotting disorders, factor VII is often given off-label after cardiac surgery for those with coagulopathies receiving blood products. Adverse effects include myocardial infarction, cardiac ischemia, supraventricular tachycardia, arterial thromboembolism, cerebral artery occlusion and ischemia, acute renal failure, and pulmonary emboli. Dosage varies. Patients receiving factor VII should be monitored carefully for thromboembolism and coagulation profile. Those with atherosclerotic disease, coagulopathies, or septicemia are at increased risk.

Aminocaproic acid
Aminocaproic acid, an antifibrinolytic agent, prevents plasminogen from binding to fibrin, interfering with the breakdown of clots. It is used in the cardiac patient with postoperative bleeding associated with fibrinolysis. Dosage is 4–5 g over 60 minutes initially and then a maintenance infusion of 1 g/hr for 8 hours or until bleeding is controlled. Adverse effects include thrombocytopenia, dysrhythmias, and thrombosis.

Abciximab

Abciximab (ReoPro) is used to prevent cardiac ischemia for patients undergoing percutaneous coronary intervention (PCI). It inhibits the aggregation of platelets. It is used with aspirin or weight-adjusted, low-dose heparin and potentiates the action of anticoagulants. However, its use with nonweight-adjusted, long-acting heparin can cause thrombocytopenia with an increased risk of hemorrhage, especially with readministration of the drug, which can induce the formation of antibodies and an allergic reaction that is characterized by anaphylaxis and thrombocytopenia, referred to as abciximab- (ReoPro-) induced coagulopathy. Because of the danger of hemorrhage, abciximab is contraindicated if there is active bleeding; a history of bleeding; a history of a cerebrovascular accident, especially within 2 years; a platelet count of less than $100,000/mm^3$; or a recent history of oral anticoagulation. Careful monitoring of platelet counts before administration and the use of weight-adjusted, low-dose heparin is important to prevent bleeding. Heparin should be discontinued after the PCI.

Heparin-rebound effect

Protamine is a polypeptide derived from salmon sperm and is used for both on- and off-pump procedures to reverse the effects of heparin. Although protamine is given at the end of surgery to reverse heparin, a heparin-rebound effect may occur after surgery, causing a recurrence of anticoagulation and increased bleeding. After cardiopulmonary bypass, some heparin remains bound to tissues and protein, and as this slowly releases, the heparin-rebound effect occurs. Additional infusions of protamine will reduce this effect. Protamine (25 mg intravenously for two doses) is indicated for postoperative mediastinal bleeding if the partial thromboplastin time is elevated. Transesophageal echocardiography is indicated if there are concerns about cardiac tamponade. Packed red blood cells are indicated for a hematocrit of less than 26 mL/dL. Desmopressin (0.3 µg/kg intravenously) is indicated for uremia or platelet dysfunction related to the use of aspirin.

Open chest wound

A cardiac surgery patient may return from the operating room with an open chest wound if an infection, such as severe mediastinitis, occurred that required debridement of tissue, leaving the wound open to heal by secondary intention. The wound may contain packing and be covered with a sterile dressing that should be changed at least every 24 hours. An open wound increases the risk of further infection, so the patient is placed on broad-spectrum antibiotics and monitored carefully. In most cases, patients are kept intubated and sedated to prevent movement until the wound can be covered with a muscle flap. Vacuum-assisted closure (negative pressure) may be used. Episodes of ischemia during surgery may cause myocardia or pulmonary edema that prevents closure of the chest wound because compression may cause cardiac tamponade. The sternum is left open until the edema subsides. A protective rubber dam is placed over the sternal opening and sutured to the skin. The dam is covered with gauze saturated in povidone-iodine and a sterile bandage.

NPWT

Application of negative pressure wound therapy (NPWT) is done after a wound is determined to be appropriate for this treatment and debridement is completed, leaving the wound tissue exposed. There are a number of different electrical suction NPWT systems, such as the vacuum-assisted closure system and the Versatile I. Several layers of paraffin or petroleum jelly (Vaseline) gauze may be placed over the heart to help prevent right ventricular rupture, but this covering is not rigid, and rupture can occur. Application steps include:
- Apply nonadherent porous foam cut to fit and completely cover the wound
- Polyurethane (hydrophobic, repelling moisture) is used for all wounds EXCEPT those that are painful, have tunneling or sinus tracts, deep trauma wounds, and wounds needing controlled growth of granulation
- Polyvinyl (hydrophilic) is used for all wounds EXCEPT deep wounds with moderate granulation, deep pressure ulcers, and flaps
- Secure foam occlusive transparent film

- Cut opening to accommodate the drainage tube in the dressing, and attach drainage tube
- Attach tube to suction canister, creating a closed system
- Set pressure as indicated
- Change dressings two to three times a week

Abnormal pulsus paradoxus

Pulsus paradoxus is a systolic blood pressure markedly lower during inhalation than exhalation. Pulsus paradoxus with a 10 mm Hg or more difference is considered abnormal and is a common sign of cardiac tamponade. A decrease in blood pressure by 10 mm Hg or less during inspiration is a normal finding, but an increased pressure difference may indicate a number of cardiopulmonary complications, including pericardial effusion, pericarditis, pulmonary embolism, cardiogenic shock, chronic obstructive pulmonary disease, asthma, and obstruction of the superior vena cava. Blood pressure should be reevaluated if pulsus paradoxus is found to ensure correct readings. Pulsus paradoxus is evaluated by finding the first systolic reading during exhalation and then decreasing blood pressure cuff readings until the systolic pressure can be heard during both cycles. A difference between the exhalation-only systolic reading and the inhalation–exhalation reading of 10 mm Hg or more is positive for pulsus paradoxus.

Myocardial stunning and hibernation

Myocardial stunning

Myocardial stunning is a period of left ventricular (LV) dysfunction occurring with reperfusion after a period (5–20 minutes) of myocardial ischemia or infarction that is too short to result in necrosis. Stunning may result from cardiopulmonary bypass or cardiac arrest. Myocardial stunning is characterized by decreased contractility, decreased tissue perfusion, and decreased levels of tissue adenine nucleotide, although coronary blood flow is normal. Symptoms usually subside over a few hours or days. The heart does not show adaptation to a chronic lack of adequate perfusion.

Myocardial hibernation

Myocardial hibernation is LV dysfunction, resulting from chronic ischemia, such as with chronic coronary disease, myocardial infarction, and heart failure. The heart adapts to the lack of adequate perfusion over time. Restoration of blood flow reverses the symptoms; however, if revascularization does not occur, permanent fibrotic changes and dysfunction can lead to congestive heart failure.

Thoracic aorta surgery patients

Dissecting aortic aneurysm

A dissecting aortic aneurysm occurs when the wall of the aorta is torn and blood flows between the layers of the wall, dilating and weakening it until it risks rupture (which has a 90% mortality). Aortic aneurysms are more than twice as common in men as women, but women have a higher mortality rate, possibly because they are often older. Different classification systems are used to describe the type and degree of dissection.

DeBakey classification uses anatomic location as the focal point:
- Type I begins in the ascending aorta but may spread to include the aortic arch and the descending aorta (60%). This is also considered a proximal lesion or Stanford type A
- Type II is restricted to the ascending aorta (10%–15%). This is also considered a proximal lesion or Stanford type A
- Type III is restricted to the descending aorta (25%–30%). This is considered a distal lesion or Stanford type B

Types I and II are thoracic, and type III is abdominal.

Surgical Procedures for Aortic Dissections and Aneurysms

Type A dissection	Resuspension or replacement of the aortic valve, resection of a tear, and insertion of an interposition graft Elephant trunk Dacron graft inserted if dissection occurs across the arch Surgery with deep hypothermic circulatory arrest (DHCA) but aortic cross-clamping not required
Type B dissection	Classic approach: resection of tear and insertion of graft Newer approach: insertion of endovascular stent Measures required to reduce spinal cord ischemia
Ascending arch aneurysm repair	Procedures: insertion of supracoronary interposition graft or valved conduit (Bentall procedure) Aortic-valve sparing procedure indicated for some patients (Marfan syndrome or bicuspid valves) Cardiopulmonary bypass required Simple cross-clamping and DHCA (central core temperature to 18°C) sometimes necessary; retrograde or antegrade cerebral perfusion with DHCA
Transverse arch aneurysm repair	May include hemiarch repair with deep hypothermic circulatory arrest (DHCA) with retrograde or antegrade cerebral perfusion or interposition graft or individual trifurcation grafts Distal arch per left thoracotomy done without cardiopulmonary bypass (CPB) or with CPB and DHCA
Descending thoracic aneurysm repair	Graft replacement of damaged aorta and reimplantation of intercostal vessels (T8–T12) with large aneurysms per left thoracotomy. Aortic cross-clamping for traditional approaches. CPB: Methods to prevent spinal cord ischemia and ischemia with aortic cross-clamping: medications, cerebral spinal fluid drainage, shunting, left-heart bypass alone, and femoro-femoral bypass, sometimes with DHCA if aortic clamping not possible Aortic cross-clamping not necessary with thoracic endovascular aortic repair; may reduce morbidity and mortality

Type A aortic dissections

The primary treatment for type A aortic dissections of the ascending aorta is surgical repair, although patients may later develop a distal aneurysm. Postoperatively, incisional bleeding is common, so status must be monitored carefully. Hypertension must be strictly controlled by antihypertensive medications to reduce blood pressure and the force of contractions, including intravenous β-blockers (esmolol, metoprolol, labetalol) with or without nitroprusside. When converted to oral medications, calcium channel blockers or angiotensin-converting enzyme inhibitors may be added. β-Blockers reduce the risk of developing further aneurysm. Because deep hypothermic circulatory arrest is required for surgery, patients must be monitored carefully for neurological impairment or stroke. Blood products should be used early if there is excessive bleeding or if coagulopathy is suspected.

Type B aortic dissections

Type B aortic dissections carry a high risk (20%–35%) of mortality with surgical repair. Complications include respiratory and renal failure and paraplegia. Renal function must be supported, and frequent neurological assessment must be carried out.

Thoracic aortic aneurysms

Thoracic aortic aneurysms are usually related to atherosclerosis but may also result from Marfan syndrome, Ehlers-Danlos disease, and connective tissue disorders. The aneurysms are often asymptomatic but may cause substernal pain, back pain, dyspnea or stridor (from pressure on the trachea), dysphagia, cough, distention of neck veins, and edema of neck and arms. Rupture usually does not allow time for emergent repair, so identifying and correcting before rupture are essential. Diagnosis is often made with x-ray or computed tomography. Cardiac catheterization and echocardiogram may also be needed. Surgery is indicated for aneurysms 6 cm or larger. Endovascular grafting is routinely done for aneurysms of the descending thoracic aorta. There is a 4% occurrence of paraplegia with thoracic aorta aneurysm repair and an increased risk of stroke.

Aneurysms of the ascending aorta

Aneurysms of the ascending aorta may result from congenital abnormalities in otherwise healthy individuals or in elderly patients with a history of hypertension, chronic lung disease, and generalized atherosclerosis. Different procedures are used, depending on which part of the ascending aorta or arch is involved. Some are repaired with an aortic cross-clamp in place with cardiopulmonary bypass and mild hypothermia, and others are cannulated for bypass (femoral or axillary artery). If extended periods of deep hypothermic circulatory arrest are required, neuroprotective procedures that increase cerebral blood flow may be used: selective antegrade cerebral perfusion or retrograde cerebral perfusion. Postoperative hypertension must be controlled, and neurologic status must be monitored. Prolonged hypothermia may result in an extended period (24 hours) of neurologic recovery. Patients usually require a temperature-controlling device postoperatively as temperature may fall. Coagulopathies and bleeding must be treated aggressively.

Descending thoracic aortic aneurysms

Repair of a descending thoracic aortic aneurysm may result in a number of complications. Excessive blood loss often requires multiple transfusions that, in turn, cause coagulopathy that requires multiple blood components and sometimes a return to surgery. Patients experience significant pain, and some require tracheostomy for prolonged mechanical ventilation. A cerebrospinal fluid (CSF) drain is placed during surgery and left in place for about 72 hours to maintain a CSF pressure of 10 mm Hg or less. The mean arterial pressure is maintained at 90 mm Hg to prevent spinal ischemia and paraplegia even though this may increase bleeding. Paraplegia may occur several days after surgery, usually because of a fall in blood pressure (BP), so treatment includes increasing BP, high-dose steroids, and replacing the CSF drain if it was removed. About 10%–15% of patients may experience renal failure as a result of impaired renal perfusion with cross-clamping of the aorta, so renal status must be carefully monitored.

Maze and coronary artery patients

Maze procdure

Cardiac rhythm disorder
The left-sided Maze procedure (Cox/Maze) is usually done with mitral valve surgery to treat atrial fibrillation (Afib) by disrupting reentrant pathways needed for Afib through development of scarring, as restoring normal sinus rhythm improves long-term survival after cardiac surgery. The left-sided Maze procedure (cut-and-sew), done with cardiopulmonary bypass, results in ablation lines around and between the right and left pulmonary veins and an additional line from

- 34 -

the inferior box lesion by the right or left inferior pulmonary vein to the mitral valve annulus. The left atrial appendage is removed, and an ablation line is placed from the appendage base to the left pulmonary veins with the base of the appendage oversewn. A variety of modifications have been made (Cox/Maze I, II, III, and IV). Cox/Maze III and IV (which uses radiofrequency ablation instead of surgical cuts externally on a beating heart) are most commonly used presently. Cox/Maze III and IV are associated with fewer recurrences of Afib. Postoperatively, patients may exhibit heart block or bradycardia because of surgical manipulation affecting the conduction system.

Atrial fibrillation

Postoperative care of patients undergoing Maze procedures is similar to those undergoing open-heart surgery. The heart rate and rhythm must be continuously monitored until both stabilize. Amiodarone is usually given at the conclusion of bypass and during the postoperative period for several months with the dosage gradually decreased as the patient establishes a normal sinus rhythm. Recurrence of atrial arrhythmias is usually treated with external cardioversion. If this is not successful, then β-blockers or digoxin may be indicated. Anticoagulation begins with heparin postoperatively when bleeding is resolved and continues with warfarin, usually for at least 3–6 months or longer if atrial arrhythmias recur or continue. The ultimate goal of treatment is to maintain a normal sinus rhythm without medications.

Coronary artery syndromes

Stable angina

Impairment of blood flow through the coronary arteries leads to ischemia of the cardiac muscle and angina pectoris, pain that may occur in the sternum, chest, neck, arms (especially the left), or back. The pain frequently occurs with crushing pain substernally, radiating down the left arm or both arms, although this type of pain is more common in men than women, whose symptoms may appear less acute and include nausea, shortness of breath, and fatigue. Elderly or diabetic patients may also have pain in the arms, no pain at all (silent ischemia), or weakness and numbness in the arms. Stable angina episodes usually last for less than 5 minutes and are fairly predictable exercise-induced episodes caused by atherosclerotic lesions blocking 75% or more of the lumen of the affected coronary artery. Precipitating events include exercise, decrease in environmental temperature, heavy eating, strong emotions (e.g., fright, anger), or exertion, including coitus. Stable angina episodes usually resolve in less than 5 minutes by decreasing activity level and administering sublingual nitroglycerin.

Unstable angina

Unstable angina (also known as preinfarction or crescendo angina) is a progression of coronary artery disease and occurs when there is a change in the pattern of stable angina. The pain may increase, may not respond to a single nitroglycerin, and may persist for 5 minutes or more. Usually pain is more frequent, lasts longer, and may occur at rest. Unstable angina may indicate rupture of an atherosclerotic plaque and the beginning of thrombus formation so it should always be treated as a medical emergency as it may indicate a myocardial infarction.

Variant angina

Variant angina (also known as Prinzmetal's angina) results from spasms of the coronary arteries, can be associated with or without atherosclerotic plaques, and is often related to smoking, alcohol, or illicit stimulants. Elevation of ST segments usually occurs with variant angina. Variant angina frequently occurs cyclically at the same time each day and often while the person is at rest. Nitroglycerin or calcium channel blockers are used for treatment.

OPCAB patients

OPCAB

Off-pump coronary artery bypass (OPCAB) applies to a bypass graft on the beating heart through a small median sternotomy with incisional length dependent on many factors. Medications (e.g., esmolol, adenosine) slow the heart rate. Special instruments and deep sutures into the pericardium are used to support the heart and place it into position so it can be accessed and stabilized more easily. The amount of manipulation depends on the areas and number of occlusions. The length of surgery varies as well but is shorter than for on-pump coronary artery bypass. OPCAB is usually preferred over minimally invasive direct coronary artery bypass if there are multiple occlusions, as all coronary arteries can be accessed with OPCAB. If marked ventricular dysfunction is present, then a ventricular assist device may be necessary to stabilize hemodynamics.

OPCAB complications

While off-pump coronary artery bypass (OPCAB) patients may have fewer and less severe complications than those receiving cardiopulmonary bypass for cardiopulmonary bypass grafts, side effects and complications are similar; the inflammatory response is lessoned with OPCAB, and patients are less likely to experience thromboembolism or cerebral hyperperfusion. About 5% of patients must be converted to on-pump coronary artery bypass (ONCAB). Patients tend to experience less bleeding, although mediastinal and pleural tubes must be assessed hourly for bleeding. Patients receive less heparin but may develop coagulopathy and protamine reactions. Serum lactate levels are lower than with ONCAB, but levels of 4 mmol/L or more pose a risk of increased morbidity. Hemodynamic status may be affected with increased pulmonary artery pressure and decreased cardiac output. Manipulation of the heart during surgery may result in decreased compliance and contractility. Incidence of stroke, atrial fibrillation, and postoperative infection is lower with OPCAB than ONCAB. Studies show that cognitive decline can occur with OPCAB as well as ONCAB. Graft occlusion can occur, especially with venous grafts.

Coronary artery bypass graft

Indications and procedure
Coronary artery bypass graft (CABG) is a surgical procedure for the treatment of angina that does not respond to medical treatment, unstable angina, a blockage of 60% or more in left main coronary artery, blockage of multiple coronary arteries that include the proximal left anterior descending artery, left ventricular dysfunction, and previous unsuccessful percutaneous cardiac interventions. The surgery is performed through a midsternal incision that exposes the heart, which is chilled and placed on cardiopulmonary bypass with blood going from the right atrium to the machine and back to the body while the aorta is clamped to keep the surgical field free of blood. Bypass grafts are sutured into place to bypass areas of occluded coronary arteries. Grafts may be obtained from various sites:
- Gastroepiploic artery (rarely used)
- Internal mammary artery (commonly used and superior to saphenous vein but procedure is more time-consuming)
- Radial artery
- Saphenous vein (commonly used, especially for emergency procedures)

Off-pump CABG

Postoperative Management with Off-pump CABG:
- Patients should be monitored for hypothermia, and temperature should be maintained

- Hemodynamic status is usually stable, and decreased cardiac output is not common
- Graft patency must be evaluated frequently as there is an increased risk for problems because of reduced visibility during surgery. Electrocardiographic changes may indicate problems. Angiography should be done with suspicion of problems
- Patients should have pacing wires with a heart rate of 80 bpm optimal initially
- β-Blockers and magnesium are usually administered in surgery to reduce the risk of atrial fibrillation.
- Patients may be fluid-overloaded and may require diuresis when they are stable
- Mediastinal bleeding is uncommon, but coagulopathy may occur; bleeding should be suspected in patients who are hemodynamically unstable

Postoperative Issues for Patients Having CABG:
- Blood pressure (BP) usually increases within a few hours of surgery, requiring a vasodilator
- Patients given β-blockers preoperatively may need pacing after cardiopulmonary bypass is discontinued
- Patients not given β-blockers preoperatively may develop tachycardia, especially younger patients or those severely anxious. Usual treatment is esmolol or metoprolol
- Patients with a hyperdynamic left ventricle may respond to vasodilators (to control hypertension) with tachycardia. In this case, systolic BP should be allowed to rise to 140 mm Hg, and then both BP and tachycardia are treated with a β-blocker
- Patients return from surgery with atrial and ventricular pacing wires. Junctional rhythm and bradycardia require pacing at 90 bpm. Atrial pacing is preferred to

atrioventricular (AV) sequential pacing with normal AV conduction. Bi-ventricular pacing (RA-BiV) is indicated for moderate-to-severe left ventricular dysfunction. Pacing in DVI or DDD modes is indicated for second- or third-degree heart block.

Postoperative Management for Patients Having CABG:
- Inotropic medications are usually started at the end of cardio-pulmonary bypass surgery and may need to be continued to maintain cardiac output. Epinephrine (1–2 µg/min) is the drug of choice but dobutamine or dopamine may be used. If response is inadequate, milrinone is given. Inotropes may be indicated for up to 12 hours with perioperative infarction or myocardial stunning
- If hemodynamic status remains unstable, an intra-aortic balloon pump (IABP) may be necessary, and if the condition persists, a ventricular assist device (VAD) may be needed
- Nitrates are used to control hypertension, usually beginning with sodium nitroprusside or nitroglycerin if signs of ischemia.
- Antiarrhythmics with lidocaine are usually given during surgery to prevent ventricular arrhythmias. Amiodarone is effective in reducing the incidence of atrial fibrillation, and β-blockers (usually metoprolol) is administered on the first postoperative day. Ventricular arrhythmias are treated with β-blockers or placement of an implantable cardioverter defibrillator. Electrocardiographic changes may indicate ischemia or myocardial infarction. Vasodilators prevent spasm of a radial graft, and antiplatelet therapy helps maintain patency of venous grafts

Harvesting grafts for CABG

A number of vessels are commonly used for coronary artery bypass grafts. In emergency situations, the saphenous vein is often harvested because it can be obtained quickly. Both the greater and lesser saphenous veins may be used. However, using veins as grafts may result in edema of the extremity from which the graft is obtained, although this risk diminishes over time. Long-term, saphenous vein grafts may exhibit atherosclerotic changes in 5–10 years. Arterial grafts remain patent for longer periods and develop atherosclerotic changes more slowly. Arteries that are used for grafts include the right and left internal mammary arteries as well as the radial artery, usually from the nondominant side. One problem with the internal mammary arteries is that they may not be long enough for multiple bypasses. Some procedures require a combination of both venous and arterial grafts.

Port access CABG

Port access coronary artery bypass graft is an alternative form of coronary artery bypass graft (CABG) that uses a number of small incisions (ports) along with cardiopulmonary bypass (CPB) and cardioplegia to do a video-assisted surgical repair. Usually three or more incisions are required, with one in the femoral area to allow access to the femoral artery for a multipurpose catheter that is threaded through to the ascending aorta to return blood from the CPB, block the aorta with a balloon, provide cardioplegic solution, and vent air. Another catheter is threaded through the femoral vein to the right atrium to carry blood to the CPB. An incision is also needed for access to the jugular vein for catheters to the pulmonary artery and the coronary sinus. One to three thoracotomy incisions are made for insertion of video imaging equipment and instruments. While the midsternal incision is avoided, multiple incisions pose the potential for possible morbidity.

Minimally invasive surgery patients

MIDCAB

Minimally invasive direct coronary artery bypass (MIDCAB) applies to a bypass graft on the beating heart through several 3–5-inch intercostal incisions, without using cardiopulmonary bypass. Different approaches include an 8–12 cm thoracotomy incision, a 5–8 cm vertical incision on one side of the sternum, or an 8–10 cm horizontal intercostal incision. Because the incision must be over the bypass area, this procedure is suitable only for bypass of one or two coronary arteries. A small portion of rib is removed to allow access to the heart, and the internal mammary artery is used for grafting. Special instruments, such as a heart stabilizer, are used to limit movement of the heart during suturing. Surgery usually takes 2–3 hours, and recovery time is decreased as patients have less pain. Because anastomosis is difficult on a beating heart, complications, such as ischemia, may occur during surgery so a cardiopulmonary bypass machine must be available. Early studies indicate that MIDCAB may provide longer lasting relief than angioplasty for single vessel occlusion.

Advantages
Minimally invasive direct coronary artery bypass (MIDCAB) is more technically difficult than the standard coronary artery bypass graft (CABG) procedure because surgery is on a beating heart and access and visibility are limited. Additionally, incomplete revascularization may result in further intervention. There are a number of advantages:

- Patients do not suffer adverse effects associated with cardiopulmonary bypass
- Recovery time is faster, and patients are discharged earlier
- Risk of infection is lower
- Use of the left or right internal mammary artery as grafts results in longer patency of the donor conduit as

they are more resistant to atherosclerosis than venous grafts

- The risk of hemorrhage and excessive blood loss is decreased
- Since there is no aortic manipulation, patients have less risk of atrial fibrillation. Intraoperative complications are decreased
- The cost is lower

Transmyocardial laser revascularization

Transmyocardial laser revascularization may be done percutaneously or through a surgical procedure with a midsternal or thoracotomy incision. Percutaneously, a fiberoptic catheter is positioned inside the ventricle and against the ischemic area. Laser bursts are used to cut 20–40 channels into but not through the myocardium. The laser burns create channels and stimulate an inflammatory response, which causes new blood vessels to form (angiogenesis), improving circulation to the myocardium and reducing ischemia and pain. If the procedure is done surgically, the catheter tip is positioned on the outside of the left ventricle rather than the inside while the heart is beating without bypass. While studies indicate that these do not affect mortality, they do reduce symptoms and increase tolerance to activity, improving the quality of life. Postoperative care for the percutaneous procedure is as for percutaneous transluminal coronary angioplasty while care for the surgical procedure is similar to that of coronary artery bypass graft.

PTCA

Percutaneous transluminal coronary angioplasty (PTCA) is an option for patients who are poor surgical candidates, who have an acute myocardial infarction, or who have uncontrolled chest pain. This procedure is usually only done to increase circulation to the myocardium by breaking through an atheroma if there is collateral circulation. Cardiac catheterization is done with a hollow catheter (sheath), usually inserted into the femoral vein or artery and fed through the vessels to the coronary arteries. When the atheroma is verified by fluoroscopy, a balloon-tipped catheter is fed over the sheath, and the balloon is inflated with a contrast agent to a specified pressure to compress the atheroma. The balloon may be inflated a number of times to ensure that residual stenosis is less than 20%. Laser angioplasty using the excimer laser is also used to vaporize plaque. Stents may be inserted during the angioplasty to maintain patency. Stents may be flexible plastic or wire mesh and are typically placed over the catheter, which is inflated to expand the stent against the arterial wall.

Complications
Cardiac catheterization and percutaneous transluminal coronary angioplasty (PTCA) pose the risk of both intraoperative and postoperative complications. During the procedure, there is a risk of damage to both the coronary artery and the heart itself. The artery may dissect, perforate, or constrict with vasospasm. A myocardial infarction may occur when a clot dislodges. Ventricular tachycardia or cardiac arrest may occur. These complications may require immediate surgical repair. Postoperative complications of cardiac catheterization and PTCA include:

- Hemorrhage or hematoma at the sheath insertion site may require pressure. The head of the bed should be flat to relieve pressure
- Thrombus or embolus may require further surgery, anticoagulation/thrombolytic treatment, or both
- Arteriovenous fistula or pseudoaneurysm from vessel trauma usually requires compression with ultrasound and surgical repair
- Retroperitoneal bleeding from an arterial tear may cause back or flank pain and may require discontinuation of anticoagulants, intravenous fluids, or blood transfusions

- Failure of angioplasty may require a repeat procedure or other surgical intervention

DCA

Directional coronary atherectomy (DCA) is removal of an atheroma from an occluded coronary artery. This procedure may be more effective than angioplasty because instead of compressing an atheroma, it shaves it away. Sometimes angioplasty is the first step in DCA if the vessel is too narrow for the DCA catheter and the last step if the tissue needs smoothing. The DCA catheter is a large balloon catheter that is usually inserted over a sheath through the femoral artery. The catheter includes an open window on one side of the balloon with a rotational cutting piston that shaves the atheroma with the plaque residue pushed inside the device for removal. The procedure may require 4–20 cuts, depending on the extent of the plaque. A similar procedure is rotational atherectomy, which uses a catheter with a diamond-chip drill at the tip, rotating at 130,000–180,000 rpms, pulverizing the atheroma into microparticles. A transluminal extraction catheter uses a motorized cutting head with a suction device for residue.

Robot-assisted coronary artery bypass

Some medical centers conduct robot-assisted coronary artery bypass, using sophisticated robotic systems, such as the da Vinci Surgical System, Computer Motion AESOP, or Zeus system. The surgeon sits at a console and uses hand grips to control manipulators that do the surgical procedure. Robotics can be used for coronary artery bypass as well as mitral valve repair. Procedures on valves and some on coronary arteries are carried out with cardiopulmonary bypass. Because access to the right ventricle is limited, it is difficult to place pacing wires. Two chest tubes are usually placed, one in the pleura and the other in an anterior mediastinal tube. Surgeons require extensive training and may require longer to conduct surgery, especially when they are inexperienced, so prolonged bypass increases the risk of compartment syndrome.

Repairing cardiac valves

There are a number of different surgical options for repair of cardiac valves.

Valvotomy/valvuloplasty is usually done through cardiac catheterization. A valvotomy/valvuloplasty may involve releasing valve leaflet adhesions that interfere with functioning of the valve. In balloon valvuloplasty, a catheter with an inflatable balloon is positioned in the stenotic valve and inflated and deflated a number of times to dilate the opening.

Closed surgical valvuloplasty involves a midsternal incision and a small hole into the heart through which the surgeon inserts a finger or dilator to repair the valve without direct visualization.

Open commissurotomy uses cardiopulmonary bypass (CPB) and an incision into the heart for direct visualization of the valve.

Annuloplasty may be done with CPB and an incision into the heart or minimally invasive procedures to repair the valve annulus (junction of valve leaflets and heart wall).

Leaflet repair is usually done with minimally invasive procedures to repair abnormal leaflets.

Aortic valve replacement

Aortic valve replacement is an open-heart procedure with cardiopulmonary bypass. Aortic valves are tricuspid (three leaflets), and repair is usually not possible, so defective valves must be replaced with either mechanical (i.e., metal, plastic, pyrolytic carbon) or biological (i.e., porcine, bovine xenografts). A newer procedure involves percutaneous aortic valve replacement with the bioprosthesis delivered arterially (femoral vein or artery) by a guidewire and under fluoroscopy.

Glycoprotein IIB/IIIA inhibitors

Glycoprotein IIB/IIIA inhibitors are drugs that are used to inhibit platelet binding and prevent clots before and after invasive cardiac procedures, such as angioplasty and stent placement. These medications are used in combination with anticoagulant drugs, such as heparin and aspirin for the following: Acute coronary syndromes (ACSs), such as unstable angina or myocardial infarctions Percutaneous coronary intervention (PCI), such as angioplasty and stent placement These medications are contraindicated in patients with a low platelet count or active bleeding.

Abciximab (ReoPro)	Used with both heparin and aspirin for ACS and PCI and affects platelet binding for 48 hours after administration
Eptifibatide (Integrilin)	Used with both heparin and aspirin for ACS and PCI and affects platelet binding for 6–8 hours after administration; not used in patients with renal problems
Tirofiban (Aggrastat)	Used with heparin for PCI patients, with reduced dosage for those with renal problems, and affects platelet blinding for only 4–8 hours after administration

Anticoagulants

Anticoagulants are used to prevent thromboemboli. All pose a risk of bleeding.

Aspirin	Often used prophylactically to prevent clots; poses less danger of bleeding than other drugs
Warfarin (Coumadin)	Blocks use of vitamin K; decreases production of clotting factors; and is used orally for patients at risk for developing blood clots, such as those with mechanical heart valves, atrial fibrillation, and clotting disorders
Heparin	The primary intravenous anticoagulant; increases the activity of antithrombin III, used for patients with myocardial infarction (MI) and those undergoing percutaneous coronary intervention (PCI) or other cardiac surgery, and monitored by activated partial thromboplastin time
Dalteparin (Fragmin) and Enoxaparin (Lovenox)	Low-molecular-weight heparins that increase activity of antithrombin III used for unstable angina, MI, and cardiac surgery
Lepirudin (Refludan) and bivalirudin (Angiomax)	Direct thrombin inhibitors used for unstable angina, PCI, and for prophylaxis and treatment for thrombosis in heparin-induced thrombocytopenia (allergic response to heparin that causes a platelet count drop of 150,000/mm^3 or less to 30%–50% of baseline, usually occurring 5–14 days after beginning heparin)

Postoperative complications of minimally invasive cardiac surgery

Dysrhythmias	Atrial fibrillation is common, decreasing cardiac output. Treatment can include diltiazem or metoprolol to control rate or amiodarone to convert rhythm. Bradycardia (often occurring with Maze procedures) may require epicardial pacing, transcutaneous pacing, or transvenous pacing. Ventricular tachycardia (VT)/ventricular fibrillation (VF) may occur early in the postoperative period, especially with electrolyte imbalance or acidosis. VT/VF may require emergent reopening of the chest.
Hypothermia	Less common in minimally invasive procedures than those requiring cardiopulmonary bypass, hypothermia may have a number of adverse effects, including coagulopathy, bleeding, hemodynamic instability, increased systemic vascular resistance, hypertension, vasoconstriction, and dysrhythmias. Shivering increases the need for oxygen, so it should be controlled with meperidine. Rewarming must be done carefully to avoid vasodilation. Volume replacement and vasopressors may be needed to prevent hypotension.
Bleeding	Postoperative bleeding is a concern for all surgical procedures, so the patient's incision, vital signs, and hemodynamic status must be monitored.

Aortic homograft

Aortic homograft uses part of a donor's aorta with the aortic valve attached to replace the recipient's faulty aortic valve and part of the ascending aorta.

Ross procedure

Ross procedure uses the patient's pulmonary artery with the pulmonary valve to replace the aortic valve and part of the aorta and then uses a donor graft to replace the pulmonary artery.

Aortic Valve Replacement

Heart block	Manipulation and surgery near the conduction system may result in heart block, especially in patients with a history of conduction disorders or aortic regurgitation. Epicardial pacing is usually used for several days after surgery. If complete heart block does not abate after a few days, then a permanent DDD pacemaker may be implanted.
Aortic regurgitation	Supraventricular rhythm should be maintained. Fluid may not improve filling pressures because of an enlarged left ventricle, but cardiac output should improve. Most patients require an α agent, such as phenylephrine or norepinephrine, to maintain blood pressure, as patients usually remain vasodilated after surgery.

Cardiac Valve Prostheses

Mechanical	Ball-and-cage or disk mechanical valves pose less risk of infection and are more durable than biologic grafts, but they have an increased risk of thromboembolism; thus, they require long-term anticoagulant therapy. These valves are commonly used for patients with renal failure, hypercalcemia, endocarditis, or sepsis.
Xenografts/ heterografts	These biologic valves are derived from pigs (porcine), cows (ovine), or horses (equine). While they do not cause thrombus formation, they are viable for only 7–10 years. They are used for women of childbearing age because of the need to avoid anticoagulation and for patients over 70 years of age, patients with a history of peptic ulcer disease, and patients who cannot tolerate long-term anticoagulation.
Homografts / allografts	Human cadaverous valves are used to replace aortic and pulmonic valves. These grafts are expensive and difficult to obtain, and viability is 10–15 years. Because they are not thrombogenic, they do not require long-term anticoagulation and are resistant to subacute bacterial endocarditis.
Autografts/ autologous valves	The pulmonic valve and part of the pulmonic artery are excised to replace an aortic valve. Because this is the patient's own tissue, long-term anticoagulation is not necessary. A homograft may be done to replace the pulmonic valve, or the patient may be left without a pulmonic valve if pulmonic vascular pressures are normal. Autografts are used for children because they grow as the child grows and are also used for women of childbearing age, patients with history of peptic ulcer disease, and patients who cannot tolerate anticoagulation. Viability is 20 years or more.

Mitral valve prolapse

Mitral valve prolapse is more common in women than men and is often asymptomatic;

however, in rare cases it can deteriorate rapidly and result in sudden death. The cause is usually genetic, with enlargement of one or both leaflets, often with a dilated annulus and elongated chordae tendineae and papillary muscles. During systole, part of one or both leaflets balloons into the atrium. If the valve becomes stretched to the point it does not close during systole, blood regurgitates from the left ventricle back into the left ventricle. Symptoms can include lightheadedness, fatigue, dyspnea, anxiety, dizziness, chest pain (unrelated to activity), and palpitations. Medical management includes eliminating smoking, caffeine, and alcohol. Antidysrhythmics, nitrates, calcium channel blockers, or β-blockers may be indicated, depending on the patient's symptoms. With advanced disease mitral valvuloplasty or replacement may be indicated.

Mitral stenosis

Mitral stenosis is caused by an autoimmune response to rheumatic fever, leading to vegetative growths on the mitral valve. It can also be caused by infective endocarditis or lupus erythematosus. Over time, the leaflets thicken and calcify, and the commissures (junctions) fuse, decreasing the size of the valve opening. Mitral stenosis reduces the flow of blood from the left atrium to the left ventricle. Pressure in the left atrium increases to overcome resistance, resulting in enlargement of the left atrium and increased pressure in the pulmonary veins and capillaries of the lung. Symptoms of exertional dyspnea usually occur when the valve is 50% occluded. There are three mechanisms by which mitral stenosis causes pulmonary hypertension:

- Increased left atrial pressure, causing a backward increase in pressure of pulmonary veins
- Hypertrophy and pulmonary artery constriction, resulting from reactive left atrial and pulmonary venous hypertension

- Thrombotic/embolic damage to pulmonary vasculature

Treatment includes drugs to control arrhythmias and hypertension, balloon valvuloplasty, percutaneous mitral balloon valvotomy (commissurotomy), and mitral valve replacement.

Mitral valve regurgitation

Mitral valve regurgitation may occur with mitral stenosis or independently. It can result from damage caused by rheumatic fever, myxomatous degeneration caused by a genetic defect in the valvular collagen, infective endocarditis, collagen vascular disease (Marfan's syndrome), or cardiomyopathy. Hypertrophy and dilation of the left ventricle may cause displacement of the leaflets and dilation of the valve. Regurgitation occurs when the mitral valve fails to close completely so that there is backflow into the left atrium from the left ventricle during systole, decreasing cardiac output. There are three phases:

- The acute phase may occur with rupture of a chordae tendineae or papillary muscle, causing sudden left ventricular flooding and overload
- The chronic compensated phase results in enlargement of the left atrium to decrease filling pressure and hypertrophy of the left ventricle to maintain stroke volume and cardiac output
- The chronic decompensated phase occurs when the left ventricle fails to compensate for the volume overload so that stroke volume and cardiac output decrease

Mitral valve surgery

Mitral stenosis
Patients are at risk for low-cardiac output syndrome because of a small left ventricle, so filling pressure must be maintained.

Pulmonary artery pressure usually falls after surgery, especially with vasodilators used during mechanical ventilation.

Right ventricular dysfunction usually requires hemodynamic support more than left ventricular dysfunction.

Ventilator failure is common because of pulmonary hypertension, fluid overload, and general poor condition. Diuresis, a plan for weaning, and nutritional support are necessary.

Most patients are dependent on diuretics and may need them for several months to prevent edema.

Mitral regurgitation
Afterload mismatch may occur with underlying left ventricular dysfunction becoming evident because of the need for more stress on the ventricular wall to eject blood. This can lead to left ventricular failure. Reducing volume overload may alleviate symptoms. Inotropic and vasodilatory agents may be necessary. Large volumes of fluid are often required because of enlargement of the left atrium and ventricle.

Considerations
Patients with a history of pulmonary hypertension often develop right ventricular (RV) dysfunction, which is treated initially with fluid administration to improve preload; however, if central venous pressure of more than 20 mm Hg does not improve, then further fluids should be avoided as this may lead to increasing dysfunction as well as left ventricular (LV) dysfunction because the septum may shift. Inotropes are indicated to support both RV and LV function (e.g., milrinone, low-dose epinephrine, dobutamine). Nesiritide may be given to decrease pulmonary arterial pressure, and pulmonary vasodilators (e.g., inhaled nitric oxide, epoprostenol, iloprost) for severe RV dysfunction. LV outflow tract obstruction may occur in some patients with small left ventricles or septal hyperplasia and may

require a return to surgery; however, some patients may respond to avoiding hypovolemia, increasing afterload, and treatment with catecholamines and β-blockers. Maintenance of sinus rhythm may require atrial or atrioventricular pacing for up to several days although long-term maintenance is unlikely with longstanding atrial fibrillation. Excess bloody drainage in a chest tube may indicate left ventricular rupture.

Aortic stenosis

Aortic stenosis is a stricture (narrowing) of the aortic valve that controls the flow of blood from the left ventricle, causing the left ventricular wall to thicken as it increases pressure to overcome the valvular resistance, increasing afterload and increasing the need for blood supply from the coronary arteries. This condition may result from a birth defect or childhood rheumatic fever and tends to worsen over the years as the heart grows.

Symptoms	Treatment
Chest pain on exertion and intolerance of exercise Heart murmur Hypotension on exertion that may be associated with sudden fainting Sudden death Tachycardia with faint pulse Poor appetite Increased risk for bacterial endocarditis and coronary insufficiency Increases mitral regurgitation and secondary pulmonary hypertension	Balloon valvuloplasty to dilate valve nonsurgically Surgical repair of valve or replacement of valve, depending on the extent of stricture Percutaneous aortic valve replacement (tri-leaflet bioprosthesis derived from equine pericardium)

Aortic valve surgery management

Hemodynamic status must be monitored carefully as it may deteriorate within 24 hours of surgery, requiring cardioversion for atrial fibrillation. If sinus rhythm is not present, atrioventricular pacing is indicated to maintain a heart rate of 90–100 bpm with left ventricular hypertrophy.

Preload should be maintained (pulmonary capillary wedge pressure > 20 mm Hg) so that the left ventricle fills adequately.

Hypertension is common within a few hours, but vasodilators may cause tachycardia with hyperdynamic cardiac status; a β-blocker (e.g., esmolol) may be effective.

With hypertrophy and a hyperdynamic left ventricle, filling pressure may increase along with decreased stroke volume and cardiac output. This is usually treated with volume infusions, but inotropes should be avoided, although milrinone or nesiritide may be used.

Aortic regurgitation

Aortic regurgitation occurs when the aortic valve fails to close properly or remain closed, resulting in reflux of blood from the aorta into the left ventricle during diastole. Causes include infective or rheumatic endocarditis, syphilis, dissecting aneurysm, congenital abnormalities, or blunt trauma. To compensate, reflex vasodilation occurs with reduced systemic vascular resistance and diastolic blood pressure. Patients exhibit low cardiac output and increased heart rate with widened pulse pressure (a characteristic sign). Patients may remain asymptomatic initially or complain of forceful heartbeat, noted in the head or neck, with arterial pulsation palpable in the carotid or temporal arteries. Over time patients develop signs of left ventricular heart failure, including orthopnea and paroxysmal nocturnal dyspnea. Patients are treated initially with a vasodilator, such as calcium channel blockers and angiotensin-converting enzyme inhibitors, but the treatment of choice is valvuloplasty or valve replacement. Postoperatively, patients may require vasodilators and inotropic agents (e.g., milrinone, dobutamine). The intra-aortic balloon pump may also be used postoperatively to maintain adequate hemodynamic status.

Pulmonic stenosis

Pulmonic stenosis is a stricture of the pulmonary blood that controls the flow of blood from the right ventricle to the lungs, resulting in right ventricular hypertrophy as the pressure increases in the right ventricle and decreased pulmonary blood flow. The condition may be asymptomatic, or symptoms may not be evident until adulthood, depending on the severity of the defect. Pulmonic stenosis may be associated with a number of other heart defects.

Symptoms	Treatment
Loud heart murmur Congestive heart murmur Mild cyanosis Cardiomegaly Angina Dyspnea Fainting Increased risk of bacterial endocarditis	Balloon valvuloplasty to separate the cusps of the valve for children. Surgical repair, including the cardiopulmonary bypass pulmonary valvotomy for older children and adults

Tricuspid valve

The tricuspid valve separates the right atrium and right ventricle and maintains forward flow of blood to the right ventricle.

Regurgitation may result from congenital abnormalities, infective diseases (e.g., rheumatic fever, endocarditis), toxic reactions, and trauma or may occur secondary to pulmonary hypertension, mitral valve disease (most common), aortic valve disease, or left heart failure. Symptoms include weakness, fatigue, peripheral edema, abnormal venous pulsations, and atrial fibrillation.

Stenosis may result from rheumatic heart disease, tumors, or endocarditis. Symptoms include peripheral venous distention, low cardiac output, fatigue, and general malaise. Surgical repair (e.g., annuloplasty, replacement) for regurgitation is usually done in conjunction with mitral valve repair. For stenosis, procedures can include open or closed commissurotomy and open valvuloplasty. However, regurgitation often develops after surgical repair.

Anticoagulation therapy

Anticoagulation therapy is indicated indefinitely for patients undergoing valve repair or replacement.
Warfarin is given for the following time periods, usually with aspirin given indefinitely.
Aortic valve replacement (tissue): 3 months (INR: 2–3) if risk factors present or aspirin, 75–100 mg, alone if no risk factors
Aortic valve replacement (mechanical): indefinitely (INR: 2–3) along with aspirin, 75–100 mg
Mitral valve repair: 3 months (INR: 2–3) OR aspirin, 75–100 mg
Mitral valve replacement (tissue): 3 months (INR: 2–3) followed by aspirin, 85–100 mg, or indefinitely with aspirin if risk factors present; with no risk factors, may be treated with aspirin alone
Mitral valve replacement (mechanical): indefinitely (INR: 2.5–3.5) with aspirin, 75–100 mg
Aortic and mitral valve replacements (tissue): 3 months (INR: 2–3) followed by aspirin, 325 mg
Aortic and mitral valve replacements (mechanical): indefinitely (INR: 3–4.5) along with aspirin, 75–100 mg

Excess anticoagulation with warfarin

Excess anticoagulation with warfarin can lead to hemorrhage, so warfarin administered after cardiac surgery should be individualized with avoidance of a loading dose. Initial dosages may range from 2.5–5 mg. Management of overanticoagulation includes:
- INR 5 or less (but above therapeutic levels) without significant bleeding: Reduce or withhold one dose until INR reaches therapeutic range
- INR 5–9 without significant bleeding: Withhold warfarin for 1–2 days until INR falls to 4 or less, OR withhold one dose of warfarin, and administer 1–2.5 mg of vitamin K orally
- INR 9 or less without significant bleeding: Withhold warfarin for 24–48 hours (until INR reaches therapeutic range), and administer vitamin K (2.5–5 mg) orally
- Any INR with severe bleeding: Withhold warfarin and administer vitamin K, 10 mg in 50 mL normal saline per intravenous infusion over 30 minutes, along with fresh frozen plasma ($\geq$ 15 mL/kg). Vitamin K may be repeated every 12 hours. Prothrombin complex concentrate (25–50 units/kg) or recombinant factor VIIa (40 μg/kg if bleeding persists

Heart valve replacement complications

Patients usually tolerate heart valve repair or replacement well, but postoperative complications can include the following:
- Cardiovascular: thromboembolism (especially if the patient received a mechanical valve), atrial dysrhythmias (most commonly atrial fibrillation), atrioventricular block, heart failure, low cardiac output, and myocardial infarction
- Renal: insufficiency
- Neurological: stroke, transient ischemic attack, and changes in mental status

- Respiratory: insufficiency, dyspnea, and orthopnea
- Bleeding: hemorrhage, sometimes requiring a return to surgery for exploration
- Infection: sternal wound infection as well as infection of the valve itself; antibiotic prophylaxis routinely given preoperatively and for 2 days postoperatively to prevent infection

Routine monitoring includes heart rate and rhythm, hemodynamic status, chest tube drainage, respiratory status, neurological status, serum electrolytes, fluid volume (avoiding reduction in preload), and pain.

Infective valve endocarditis

Infective valve endocarditis may occur in native valves and prosthetic valves, generally affecting the mitral, tricuspid, or aortic valve. Indications may include fever, heart murmur, and hemodynamic instability. Signs of heart failure may occur. Vegetations, ulcerations, and abscesses may occur. Indications for surgery vary, according to the degree of involvement, the spread of infection, the infective agent, and the persistence and size of vegetations. During surgery, all infected tissue must be removed:

- Aortic valve: Replacement may be with a homograft (preferred if possible), tissue, or mechanical valves
- Tricuspid valve: Repair is preferred, especially for high-risk patients, such as drug abusers. In some cases valvulectomy (if no pulmonary hypertension) or valve replacement may be indicated
- Mitral valve: Leaflet repair may be sufficient with early intervention, although more severe disease requires valve replacement
- Antibiotics are usually given for 6 weeks perioperatively, but when cultures taken during surgery show organisms, antibiotics are usually continued for 6 weeks postoperatively

Radial artery as an alternate arterial conduit

Radical artery

The radial artery has become increasingly popular as an arterial graft because of its long duration of patency; however, the adequacy of collateral vessels and circulation to the hand by the ulnar artery must be assessed preoperatively by the Allen test and Doppler flow measurements. With the Allen test, flushing that takes 6 seconds or more is considered a contraindication for use of the radial artery. Other contraindications include peripheral vascular disease, Raynaud's, stroke, or traumatic injury on the graft side. After harvesting, surgeons may place a drain, which is usually removed when drainage decreases to less than 20 mL/8 hr. A compression dressing is usually left in place for 24 hours. The wound should be assessed for drainage, capillary refill time, indications of infection and hematoma, temperature, and ulnar artery pulse, including evaluating the 6 Ps (pain, pulselessness, pallor, paresthesia, paralysis, polar/cold). Weakness and numbness may persist for 6 months or less. Patients receive calcium channel blockers (e.g., diltiazem) during surgery and for 6 months postoperatively. Cellulitis may develop but usually responds to antibiotics.

Pulmonary

Acute respiratory failure

Phrenic nerve damage

The phrenic nerve controls the action of the diaphragm and is essential to breathing. If the phrenic nerve is injured, this can cause unilateral or bilateral diaphragmatic dysfunction (paralysis). Injury (occurring in 1%–30% of cardiac surgery patients) may result from iced slush used for myocardial

- 48 -

protection during cardioplegic arrest. Damage to the nerve may also occur with harvesting of the left internal mammary artery or other surgical trauma. Unilateral injury is most common and usually does not severely impair ventilation, although lower lobe atelectasis, especially on the left, may occur. Symptoms include paradoxical movement of the diaphragm, nocturnal orthopnea, or dyspnea on exertion. Bilateral injuries may result in a longer duration of mechanical ventilation, difficulty weaning, prolonged nocturnal respiratory insufficiency, and in some cases acute respiratory failure. Plication of the diaphragm may be necessary to improve pulmonary function if the patient's respirations are severely compromised. Diagnosis is by chest x-ray, fluoroscopy, spirometry, nerve conduction studies, or ultrasound.

Acute respiratory failure symptoms

The symptoms of acute respiratory failure include:
- Tachypnea
- Tachycardia
- Anxiety and restlessness

In cardiac surgery patients, acute respiratory failure may be caused by bilateral phrenic nerve injury and diaphragmatic paralysis. Early signs may include difficulty weaning from the ventilator. After removal from ventilation, signs and symptoms include changes in the depth and pattern of respirations with flaring nares, sternal retractions, expiratory grunting, wheezing, and extended expiration as the body tries to compensate for hypoxemia and increasing levels of carbon dioxide. Cyanosis may be evident. Central nervous depression, with alterations in consciousness, occurs with decreased perfusion to the brain. As the hypoxemia worsens, cardiac arrhythmias, including bradycardia, may occur with either hypotension or hypertension. Dyspnea becomes more pronounced with depressed respirations. Eventually stupor, coma, and

death can occur if the condition is not reversed.

Hypoxemic respiratory failure

Hypoxemic respiratory failure occurs suddenly when gaseous exchange of oxygen for carbon dioxide cannot keep up with demand for oxygen or the production of carbon dioxide.
- Partial pressure of oxygen (PaO_2) < 60 mm Hg
- Partial pressure of carbon dioxide ($PaCO_2$) > 40 mm Hg
- Arterial pH < 7.35

Hypoxemic respiratory failure can be the result of low-inhaled oxygen, as at high elevations or with smoke inhalation. The following ventilatory mechanisms may be involved:
- Alveolar hypotension
- Ventilation–perfusion mismatch (the most common cause)
- Intrapulmonary shunts
- Diffusion impairment

Hypercapnic respiratory failure

Hypercapnic respiratory failure results from an increase in $PaCO_2$ (> 45–50 mm Hg) associated with respiratory acidosis and may include the following:
- Reduction in minute ventilation, total volume of gas ventilated in 1 minute, often related to neurological, muscle or chest-wall disorders, drug overdoses, or obstruction of upper airway
- Increased dead space with wasted ventilation (related to lung disease or disorders of the chest wall, such as scoliosis)
- Increased production of carbon dioxide (usually related to infection, burns, or other causes of hypermetabolism)

IRV

Inspiratory reserve volume (IRV) is the amount of air that can be taken into the lungs with forced inhalation after a normal resting inspiratory effort.

ERV

Expiratory reserve volume (ERV), conversely, is the amount of air that can be exhaled through forced exhalation after a normal resting exhalation.

RV

Residual volume (RV) is the volume of air remaining in the lungs after ERV is completed.

Vt

Tidal volume (Vt) is the volume of air that is inhaled or exhaled in a single breath.

IC

Inspiratory capacity (IC) is the maximum volume of air that can be inhaled from a resting exhalation. It can be calculated by the equation Vt + IRV = IC, or it can be measured directly.

FRC

Functional residual capacity (FRC) is the combination of the expiratory reserve volume and the residual volume. This is defined as the volume of air in the lungs at resting tidal exhalation.

VC

Vital capacity (VC) is the maximum amount of air that can be forced out of the lungs following a maximum inhalation. It is defined as IRV + Vt + ERV = VC.

TLC

Total lung capacity (TLC) is the total sum of all of the air that the lungs can contain. It is defined as IRV + Vt + ERV + RV = TLC.

Alveolar hypoventilation

Alveolar hypoventilation occurs when the effectiveness of alveolar gas exchange reduces so the partial pressures of oxygen and carbon dioxide both increase. The failure to eliminate carbon dioxide displaces oxygen in the alveolar sacs.

Physiologic shunting

Physiologic shunting is venous blood in the lung bypassing the alveoli and re-entering the arterial system. This normally occurs with 2%–3% of venous blood but may increase with alveolar congestion related to pulmonary edema, atelectasis, or other disorder.

Intrapulmonary shunting

Intrapulmonary shunting involves alveolar perfusion without ventilation, so the oxygenated blood reaches the alveolus but cannot exchange for carbon dioxide because the alveolus is damaged or diseased.

Refractory hypoxemia

Refractory hypoxemia occurs when there is so much loss of alveoli that oxygen administration is unable to correct the hypoxemia.

Dead space

Dead space occurs when a well-ventilated alveolus cannot be perfused because of blockage by an embolus, capillary compression, or other damage.

Ventilation–perfusion mismatch

Ventilation–perfusion mismatch (V/Q) occurs when well-ventilated alveoli lack adequate perfusion (creating partial dead space) or poorly ventilated alveoli have adequate perfusion (creating partial shunts).

Respiratory failure

Respiratory failure must be treated immediately before severe hypoxemia causes irreversible damage to vital organs.

Identifying and treating the underlying cause should be done immediately because emergency medications or surgery may be indicated. Medical treatments vary widely, depending on the cause; for example, cardiopulmonary structural defects may require surgical repair; pulmonary edema may require diuresis; inhaled objects may require surgical removal; and infections may require aggressive antimicrobials.

Intravenous lines/central lines are inserted for testing, fluids, and medications.

Oxygen therapy should be initiated to attempt to reverse hypoxemia; however, if refractory hypoxemia occurs, then oxygen therapy alone will not suffice. Oxygen levels must be titrated carefully.

Intubation and mechanical ventilation are frequently required to maintain adequate ventilation and oxygenation. Positive end expiratory pressure may be necessary with refractory hypoxemia and collapsed alveoli.

Respiratory status must be monitored constantly, including arterial blood gases and vital signs.

ALI and ARDS

Pathophysiology
Acute lung injury (ALI) comprises a syndrome of respiratory distress culminating in acute respiratory distress syndrome (ARDS), a rare complication of cardiac surgery. ALI and ARDS usually occur more than 24 hours postoperatively. ARDS is characterized by damage to the vascular endothelium and an increase in the permeability of the alveolar–capillary membrane when damage to the lung results from toxic substances (e.g., gastric fluids, bacteria, chemicals, toxins emitted by neutrophils as part of the inflammatory-mediated response); these substances reduce surfactant and cause pulmonary edema as the alveoli fill with blood and protein-rich fluid and then collapse. Atelectasis with hyperinflation and areas of normal tissue occur as the lungs "stiffen." The fluid in the alveoli becomes a medium for infection. Because there is neither adequate ventilation nor perfusion, the result is increasing hypoxemia and tachypnea as the body tries to compensate to maintain a normal partial pressure of carbon dioxide. Untreated, the condition results in respiratory failure, multiorgan failure, and a mortality rate of 15%–70% when it occurs as a complication of cardiac surgery.

ARDS

Symptoms
Patients presenting with acute respiratory distress syndrome may initially present with only mild tachypnea, but more serious symptoms develop as respiratory function becomes more compromised:
- Crackling rales or wheezing may be heard throughout the lungs
- A decrease in pulmonary compliance (lung volume), referred to as "baby lung," results in increasing tachypnea with expiratory grunting
- Cyanosis may develop with characteristic blue discoloration of lips and skin mottling
- Hypotension and tachycardia may occur
- Symptoms associated with volume overload are missing (e.g., third heart sound, jugular venous distention)

- 51 -

- Respiratory alkalosis is often an early sign but is replaced as the disease progresses with hypercarbia and respiratory acidosis
- X-ray studies may be normal at first but then show diffuse infiltrates in both lungs, but the heart and vessels appear normal

Management

The management of acute respiratory distress syndrome (ARDS) involves providing adequate gas exchange and preventing further damage to the lung from forced ventilation. Treatment includes the following: Oxygen therapy by nasal prongs/cannula or mask may be sufficient in mild cases to maintain oxygen saturation (SpO_2) above 90%. Oxygen should be administered at 100% because of the mismatch between ventilation (V) and perfusion (Q), which can result in hypoxia on position change. Endotracheal intubation may be needed if SpO_2 falls or carbon dioxide levels rise. Mechanical ventilation with lower tidal volumes (6 mL/kg) or high-frequency oscillatory ventilation to maintain SpO_2 over 90%.

Inhaled nitric oxide may be prescribed for pulmonary hypertension.

Prophylactic antibiotics are not indicated. Steroids may increase survival rates if given later in treatment if ARDS has not resolved within a week.

Pulmonary dysfunction

Pulmonary dysfunction can result from many factors related to cardiac surgery.

General anesthesia and anesthetic agents, such as paralytic agents, result in decreased respiratory drive and impairment of the diaphragm and intercostal muscles. The supine position causes the chest wall to relax and changes in compliance.

Cardiopulmonary bypass may result in pulmonary edema, interstitial pulmonary edema, and adult respiratory distress syndrome because of an inflammatory response and capillary leak. Inadequate ventilation of alveoli may result in atelectasis. The phrenic nerve injury from cooling may cause diaphragmatic paralysis.

Sternotomy or thoracotomy may result in pain and splinting that impairs respirations.

Internal mammary artery harvesting may cause impaired chest wall compliance because of incision into the pleura.

Preexisting conditions, such as pulmonary disease or obesity, may further impair respirations.

Habits, such as smoking, may cause increased bronchospasm and muscle weakness.

Mechanical ventilation for over 48 hours increases the risk of pneumonia.

Air leak syndrome

Air leak syndrome may occur spontaneously or secondary to some type of trauma (e.g., accidental, mechanical, iatrogenic) or disease. As pressure increases inside the alveoli, the alveolar wall pulls away from the perivascular sheath and subsequent alveolar rupture allows air to follow the perivascular planes and flow into adjacent areas. There are two categories:

- Pneumothorax: Air is in the pleural space
- Barotrauma/volutrauma: Air is in the interstitial space

Pneumoperitoneum

Pneumoperitoneum means air is in the peritoneal area, including the abdomen.

Pneumomediastinum

Pneumomediastinum means air is in the mediastinal area between the lungs.

Retrosternal and neck pain, dyspnea, and slight neck edema indicate pneumomediastinum.

Pneumopericardium

Pneumopericardium means air is in the pericardial sac.

Subcutaneous emphysema

Subcutaneous emphysema means air is in the subcutaneous tissue planes of the chest wall.

Pulmonary interstitial emphysema

Pulmonary interstitial emphysema means air is trapped in the interstitium between the alveoli.

Hamman's sign

Hamman's sign, a precordial rasping sound heard on auscultation during a heartbeat as the heart moves against tissues filled with air, is an indication of both pneumomediastinum and pneumopericardium but is not generally present with pneumothorax or cardiac tamponade.

Pneumothorax

Pneumothorax occurs when there is a leak of air into the pleural space, resulting in complete or partial collapse of a lung, because of direct injury, central venous cannulation, or barotrauma. Pneumonia-thorax usually occurs early after cardiac surgery. Tension pneumo-thorax often occurs with mechanical ventilation, usually after right pneumothorax caused by an accidental cut into the right pleura.

Symptoms:
- Vary widely, depending on the cause and degree of the pneumothorax and whether or not there is underlying disease:
  - Acute pleuritic pain (95%), usually on the affected side
  - Decreased breath sounds
  - Tension pneumothorax: tracheal deviation, distended neck veins, and hemodynamic compromise

Diagnosis:
- Clinical findings: deteriorating arterial blood gasses, hemodynamic instability, & increase in peak inspiratory pressure with ventilation
- Radiograph: 6-foot upright posterior–anterior
- Ultrasound to attempt to detect traumatic pneumothorax

Treatment:
- Chest-tube thoracostomy with underwater seal drainage (most common treatment)
- Tension pneumothorax: immediate needle decompression and chest tube thoracostomy
- Small pneumothorax: oxygen administration (3–4 L/min) and observation for 3–6 hours

Pleural effusion

Pleural effusion is common after cardiac surgery, occurring in 41%–87% of patients; it appears as an opacity on a radiograph. A pleural effusion usually arises within the first 24 hours, especially if chest tubes are not placed in the most dependent part of the pleural space. Common indications include dyspnea, dry nonproductive cough, chest pain, and orthopnea, although small effusions (< 500 mL) may remain asymptomatic. Pleural effusions are most common on the left but may occur bilaterally. Small pleural effusions resolve over time, but large pleural effusions (> 50% of lung) may require thoracentesis (often with ultrasound guidance) to drain fluid and relieve dyspnea. Correct positioning of chest tubes during surgery can help reduce the incidence of pleural effusions. Large pleural effusions may result in cardiac tamponade and atrial or ventricular diastolic collapse.

Chylothorax

In some cases, interruption of the lymphatic system of the thoracic duct in the left proximal mediastinum during mobilization of the left internal mammary artery results in chylothorax, an expanding pleural effusion with milky fluid, related to dietary fat.

Chylothorax may occur after chest tube removal with the enlarging pleural effusion noted on radiograph. Chyle is found in the pleural fluid, which contains increased levels of lymphocytes and triglycerides (> 110 mg/dL). The drainage may appear to be purulent, so chyle must be verified by laboratory analysis. Treatment includes chest tube drainage, nonfat diet, and medium-chain triglycerides. Octreotide, 100 μg, may be given subcutaneously every 8 hours to seal the leak if it does not clear within a few days. In some cases, thoracoscopic repair may be necessary

Hemothorax

Hemothorax occurs with bleeding into the pleural space. Draining of mediastinal blood into the pleural space after cardiac surgery may result in a hemothorax. Additionally, a hemothorax may result from vascular injury related to central venous pressure catheters. A small bleed may be self-limiting and seal, but a large tear or excessive bleeding can result in massive blood loss, followed quickly by hypovolemic shock. The pressure from the blood may result in an inability of the lung to ventilate and a mediastinal shift. Often a hemothorax occurs with a pneumothorax. Further symptoms include severe respiratory distress, decreased breath sounds, and dullness on auscultation. Treatment includes controlling bleeding, placement of a chest tube, or ensuring patency to drain the hemothorax; with large volumes, the pressure may be preventing exsanguination, which can

occur abruptly as the blood drains and pressure is reduced. Autotransfusion may be used to replace blood lost.

Atelectasis

Atelectasis, especially of the left lower lobe, occurs postoperatively in up to 70% of patients who have had cardiac surgery. Right-sided atelectasis most commonly occurs with fluid overload. Direct topical hypothermia (cold cardioplegia) to the heart can damage the left phrenic nerve and cause paresis or paralysis of the diaphragm, resulting in increased incidence of left lower lobe atelectasis. Harvesting of the internal thoracic artery is also associated with high rates of pleural effusion and atelectasis. Additionally, single lung ventilation and collapsing of one lung as part of the intraoperative procedure increases risks. Symptoms may be evident in the immediate postoperative period and include splinting, decreased ventilation, decreased oxygen saturation, and increased heart rate. Deep breathing, use of an incentive spirometer, intermittent positive pressure breathing treatments, and early ambulation may all help to prevent atelectasis.

Acute pulmonary embolism

Overview
Acute pulmonary embolism occurs when a pulmonary artery or arteriole is blocked by a blood clot originating in the venous system or the right heart. While most pulmonary emboli are from thrombus formation, other causes may be air, fat, or septic embolus (from bacterial invasion of a thrombus). After cardiac surgery, most incidences are associated with deep venous thrombosis of the lower extremities. Other originating sites are the pelvic veins and the right atrium. Causes include stasis related to damage to the endothelial wall and changes in blood coagulation factors. Atrial fibrillation poses a serious risk because blood pools in the right atrium, forming clots that travel directly through the right ventricle to the lungs. The

obstruction of the artery or arteriole causes an increase in alveolar dead space in which there is ventilation but impairment of gas exchange because of the ventilation–perfusion mismatching or intrapulmonary shunting. This results in hypoxia, hypercapnia, and the release of mediators that cause bronchoconstriction. If more than 50% of the vascular bed becomes excluded, pulmonary hypertension occurs.

<u>Symptoms and diagnostic tests</u>
Clinical manifestations of acute pulmonary embolism (PE) vary, according to the size of the embolus and the area of occlusion.

Symptoms	Diagnostic Tests
Dyspnea with tachypnea Tachycardia Anxiety and restlessness Chest pain Fever Rales Cough (sometimes with hemoptysis) Hemodynamic instability	Arterial blood gas analysis may show hypoxemia (decreased partial pressure of oxygen), hypocarbia (decreased partial pressure of carbon dioxide), and respiratory alkalosis (increased pH). D-dimer will show elevation with PE. Electrocardiogram may show sinus tachycardia or other abnormalities. Echocardiogram can show emboli in the central arteries and can assess the hemodynamic status of the right side of the heart. Chest x-ray is of minimal value. Spiral computed tomography may provide a definitive diagnosis. Ventilation–perfusion scintigraphy can confirm the diagnosis. Pulmonary angiograms also can confirm the diagnosis.

<u>Medical management</u>
Medical management of pulmonary embolism starts with preventive measures for those at risk, including leg exercises, elastic compression stockings, and anticoagulation therapy (warfarin [Coumadin]). Most pulmonary emboli present as medical emergencies, so the immediate task is to stabilize the patient. Medical management may include the following:

- Oxygen to relieve hypoxemia
- Intravenous infusions
- Dobutamine (Dobutrex) or dopamine (Intropin) to relieve hypotension
- Cardiac monitoring for dysrhythmias
- Medications as indicated: digitalis glycosides, diuretic, and antiarrhythmics
- Intubation and mechanical ventilation
- Analgesia (morphine sulfate) or sedation to relieve anxiety
- Anticoagulants to prevent recurrence, including heparin and warfarin (Coumadin) but will not dissolve clots already present
- Placement of percutaneous venous filter (Greenfield) in the inferior vena cava to prevent further emboli from entering the lungs if anticoagulation therapy is contraindicated
- Thrombolytic therapy, recombinant tissue-type plasminogen activator or streptokinase, for those severely compromised with limited success; a danger of bleeding

Hematology

Inflammatory response

Hyperdynamic state without infection

A hyperdynamic state without documented infection may occur after cardiac surgery, especially after prolonged extracorporeal circulation (ECC). Symptoms usually occur within 6 hours of ECC. An immune (cellular and humoral) response occurs from blood contact with the ECC unit. Proinflammatory cytokines are released. The triad of characteristics associated with the hyperdynamic state includes the following:

- Temperature elevation (> 38°C) [the best indicator]

- Increased cardiac index over 3.5 mL/min/m²
- Systemic vascular resistance index less than 1600 dynes/sec/cm⁻⁵

Patients with coronary artery surgery are at increased risk over those with valve surgery, perhaps because the length of time on cardiopulmonary bypass for valvular surgery is decreased. Typically, patients exhibit vasodilation and increased cardiac output as an inflammatory response, often resulting in hypotension leading to shock. Treatment may include fluid resuscitation and vasopressors. Other causes of the hyperdynamic state can include hyperthyroidism, Paget's disease, and beriberi.

Anemia

Anemia is common with cardiac surgery because of hemodilution associated with cardiopulmonary bypass (CPB). Hematocrit levels are usually maintained at about 20% during CPB and at 22%–24% in the postoperative period, although patients of advanced age may require transfusions to increase hematocrit if they experience marked fatigue or weakness, electrocardiographic abnormalities, or marked tachycardia. Usually postoperative diuresis increases the hematocrit slowly, but the level may remain depressed as fluid moves from the blood into extracellular tissues. Additional extracorporeal circulation damages red blood cells, shortening their lifespans, and about 30% of red blood cells received by transfusion are lost within 24 hours. Patients with a hematocrit of less than 30% at the time of discharge should receive iron supplementation with ferrous sulfate or ferrous gluconate (300 mg three times daily for 4 weeks), although this may not be necessary if the patient has received multiple transfusions because of iron retained from hemolysis.

Anaphylaxis

Anaphylaxis syndrome

Anaphylaxis syndrome is a sudden acute systemic immunoglobulin E (IgE)/G (IgG) or non-immunoglobulin E (non-IgE/non-IgG) inflammatory response affecting the cardiopulmonary and other systems.

IgE-mediated or IgG response (anaphylactic shock) is an antibody–antigen reaction against an allergen, such as milk, peanuts, latex, insect bites, or fish (and fish-derived medications, such as protamine). This is the most common type.

Non–IgE-/non–IgG-mediated response (anaphylactoid reaction) is a systemic reaction to infection, exercise, radio contrast material, or other triggers. While the response is almost identical to the other type, it does not involve IgE/IgG.

Typically, with IgE-mediated response, an antigen triggers release of substances, such as histamine and prostaglandins, which affect the skin and the cardiopulmonary and gastrointestinal systems. Histamine causes initial erythema and edema by inducing vasodilation. Each time the person has contact with the antigen, more antibodies form in response, so allergic reactions worsen with each contact. In some cases, initial reactions may be mild, but subsequent contact can cause severe life-threatening response.

Protamine anaphylactic reaction

Type I
Protamine sulfate, a heparin antagonist, is comprised of strongly basic proteins derived from salmon sperm and some other fish, so allergies to fish can put the patient at risk for protamine anaphylactic reaction. Skin testing and prophylaxis with histamine blockers and steroids have not proven of value. There are three different types of reactions.

Hypotension may occur if protamine is given too rapidly (within 3 minutes) of discontinuation of cardio-pulmonary bypass. This histamine-related response decreases systemic vascular resistance and pulmonary vascular resistance. This reaction is reversible with administration of an α agent. Protamine should be administered over 10–15 minutes to avoid this reaction. This reaction is common in diabetics who take protamine-containing insulin.

Type II

Protamine sulfate, a heparin antagonist, is comprised of strongly basic proteins derived from salmon sperm and some other fish, so allergies to fish can put the patient at risk for protamine anaphylactic reaction. Skin testing and prophylaxis with histamine blockers and steroids have not proven of value. There are three different types of reactions.

Reactions may be anaphylactic or anaphylactoid:

- IIA: Anaphylactic (IgE or IgG) reaction results in a systemic capillary leak and hypotension with pulmonary edema, usually within 10–20 minutes of administration
- IIB: Immediate anaphylactoid reaction is seen
- IIC: Reaction is delayed for 20 minutes or more. The patient may exhibit wheezing, pulmonary edema (noncardiogenic) related to capillary leak, hypotension, and hypovolemia

Type III

Type III Protamine Anaphylactic Reaction

Signs and Symptoms	Treatment
Sudden onset of weakness, dizziness, confusion	Calcium chloride, 500 mg intravenously (IV), to increase systemic vascular resistance (SVR)
Urticaria	
Increased permeability of vascular system and loss of vascular tone	α agents: phenylephrine/norepinephrine to increase SVR
Peripheral dilation with severe hypotension, leading to shock	
Laryngospasm/bronchospasm with obstruction of airway, causing dyspnea and wheezing	β agents: low-dose epinephrine, milrinone, inamrinone, and dobutamine to decrease pulmonary resistance
Increased pulmonary artery pressure	
Nausea, vomiting, and diarrhea	Nitrates: nitroglycerin to decrease preload and pulmonary pressures
Seizures, coma, and death	

Neurology/Gastrointestinal

Type I neurological deficits

Type I neurological deficits associated with cardiac surgery include those with high morbidity: major focal neurological deficits, strokes, transient ischemic attacks, stupor, and coma. These occur in over 3% of cardiac surgery patients and result in a 21% mortality rate. Patients with type I neurological deficits tend to have an increased length of hospitalization and increased need for support after discharge. Risk factors include age over 70 years, with a history of pulmonary disease, hypertension, moderate-to-severe proximal aortic atherosclerosis, left main coronary stenosis, diabetes mellitus, or unstable angina. Other surgical risk factors include use of an intra-aortic balloon pump or a left ventricular assist device and perioperative hypoperfusion. Aortic lesions are of special concern as manipulation of the aorta during surgery may result in emboli, so risk increases with the number of aortic anastomoses.

Type II neurological deficits

Type II neurological deficits associated with cardiac surgery include changes in mental status, confusion, loss of memory, agitation, disorientation, and seizures. Type II deficits are more common than the more severe type I deficits and may be more difficult to diagnose because the symptoms are more subtle and may be overlooked as simply a response to anesthesia or analgesia. While drugs may exacerbate symptoms, they persist even after the drugs are discontinued. Studies show that over half of patients undergoing coronary artery bypass graft experience type II neurological deficits. Risk factors for type II deficits include age over 70 years and a history of pulmonary disease, hypertension, or heart failure as well as a history of alcoholism. Other surgical risk factors include

development of postoperative dysrhythmias, history of previous cardiac surgery, and episodes of hypoperfusion or hypotension.

Encephalopathy

Cerebral hypoxia

Cerebral hypoxia (hypoxic encephalopathy) occurs when the oxygen supply to the brain is decreased. If hypoxia is mild, the brain compensates by increasing cerebral blood flow, but it can only double in volume and cannot compensate for severe hypoxic conditions. Hypoxia may be the result of insufficient oxygen in the environment, inadequate exchange at the alveolar level of the lungs, or inadequate circulation to the brain. Brain cells may begin dying within 5 minutes if deprived of adequate oxygenation, so any condition or trauma that interferes with oxygenation can result in brain damage.

- Near-drowning
- Asphyxia
- Cardiac arrest
- High altitude sickness
- Carbon monoxide
- Diseases that interfere with respiration, such as myasthenia gravis and amyotrophic lateral sclerosis
- Anesthesia complications

Symptoms include increasing neurological deficits, depending on the degree and area of damage, with changes in mentation that range from confusion to coma. Prompt identification of the cause and an increase in perfusion to the brain are critical for survival.

Anoxic encephalopathy

Anoxic encephalopathy, resulting from complete lack of oxygen to the brain, can occur with cardiac arrest, head trauma, asphyxia, increasing intracranial pressure, fat embolism, status epilepticus, and severe cerebral atherosclerosis. Biochemical changes occur in the brain within 5 minutes without oxygenation.

Assessment includes the following:
- Level of consciousness: Verbal stimuli, shaking patient, and digital supraorbital pressure are used to elicit a response
- Motor activity: Brainstem damage: flaccidity and areflexia
- Mid-brain and upper pons damage: extensor posturing
- Hemispheric damage: flexor posturing
- Eyes: Pupillary response and elicited eye movements if absent indicate severe damage
- Papilledema may occur after cardiac arrest without an increase in intracranial pressure.
- Horizontal movement of the eyes can persist with damage to the frontal or occipital areas if the midbrain and pons are intact
- Imaging: Magnetic resonance imaging provides better early information than computed tomography. Electroencephalogram shows cortical and epileptic activity.

Treatment depends on the causes, but reestablishing circulation is primary. After cardiac arrest, hypothermia (32°C–34°C) with neuromuscular blockade should be initiated quickly with rewarming after 24 hours to reduce cerebral damage.

Metabolic encephalopathy

Metabolic encephalopathy (hepatic encephalopathy) is damage to the brain resulting from a disturbance in metabolism, primarily hepatic failure to remove toxins from the blood. There may be impairment in cerebral blood flow, cerebral edema, or increased intracranial pressure. It can occur as the result of ingestion of drugs or toxins, which can have a direct toxic affect on neurons but can also occur with liver disease, especially when stressed by co-morbidities, such as hemorrhage, hypoxemia, surgery, trauma, renal failure with dialysis, or electrolyte imbalances. Symptoms may vary:

- Irritability and agitation
- Alterations in consciousness
- Dysphonia
- Lack of coordination and spasticity
- Seizures, commonly the presenting symptom
- Disorientation progressing to coma

Prompt diagnosis is important because the condition may be reversible if underlying causes are identified and treated before permanent neuronal damage occurs. Treatment varies, according to the underlying cause.

Delirium

Delirium is an acute sudden change in consciousness, characterized by a reduced ability to focus or sustain attention, language, memory disturbance, disorientation, confusion, audiovisual hallucinations, sleep disturbance, agitation, and psychomotor activity disorder. Delirium differs from disorders with similar symptoms in that it is fluctuating. Delirium is the most common neurological disorder associated with cardiac surgery, occurring in 3%–7% of patients with onset of symptoms most common 48–72 hours after surgery. Risk factors include preexisting psychological disorders, alcohol abuse, left ventricular ejection fraction less than 30%, 65 years of age or older, cerebral artery disease, emergent surgery, circulatory arrest over 30 minutes, electrolyte imbalances, and hypothermia (< 25°C). Medications (e.g., ß-blockers, calcium channel blockers, angiotensin-converting enzyme inhibitors, diuretics, antiarrhythmic drugs, statins) also increase the risk. Treatment includes the following:
- Identifying and treating underlying cause
- Providing supportive measures, such a reducing sensory input and promoting sleep
- Treating symptoms, usually with haloperidol (initial dose of 1–2 mg

every 2–4 hours), lorazepam, or trazodone
- Barbiturates should be avoided, and benzodiazepine should be restricted to those going through alcohol withdrawal

Confusion Assessment Method

The Confusion Assessment Method is used to assess the development of delirium and is intended for those without psychiatric training to help differentiate delirium from other types of confusion. The tool covers nine factors. Some factors have a range of possibilities, and others are rated only as to whether the characteristic is present, not present, uncertain, or not applicable. The tool provides room to describe abnormal behavior. Factors indicative of delirium include the following:
- Onset: acute change in mental status
- Attention: inattentive, stable, or fluctuating
- Thinking: disorganized, rambling conversation, switching topics, or illogical
- Level of consciousness: altered, ranging from alert to coma
- Orientation: disoriented (person, place, time)
- Memory: impaired
- Perceptual disturbances: hallucinations or illusions
- Psychomotor abnormalities: agitation (tapping, picking, moving) or retardation (staring, not moving)
- Sleep–wake cycle: awake at night and sleepy in the daytime

This tool indicates delirium if there is an acute onset with fluctuating inattention and disorganized thinking or altered level of consciousness.

Postoperative impaired cognition

Impaired cognition is very common after both on-pump and off-pump cardiac procedures with estimates ranging as high as 50%–80%. Symptoms include forgetfulness, short attention span, impaired memory, inability to think of appropriate words, and reduced psychomotor function. Risk factors include preexisting cerebrovascular disease, diabetes, and advanced age. Impaired cognition is most pronounced in those with preoperative cognitive abnormalities. Early impaired cognition is believed to be related to cerebral microembolization and hypoperfusion or an inflammatory response to cardiopulmonary bypass, which may be reversible. Other possible causes include intraoperative hyperthermia and hyperglycemia. Delayed impaired cognition is more likely related to preexisting cerebrovascular disease and is more likely to be permanent. Studies indicate that about 53% of patients exhibit impaired cognition at discharge with improvement at 6 months (24%) and then a decline with increasing rates (42%) of impaired cognition by 5 years, but some of the increase may be attributed to aging.

Neuroprotective strategies

Neuroprotective strategies should begin with careful screening of patients to determine those at increased risk. Patients who undergo cardiopulmonary bypass (CPB) should be screened for *N*-methyl-D-aspartate, a receptor antibody that is associated with an 18-fold increase in postoperative neurological deficit. Other neuroprotective strategies include the following:
- Using ultrasound or transesophageal, echocardiography to avoid atheromas
- Evaluating carotid disease preoperatively
- Administering statins preoperatively
- Using an internal mammary artery Y graft for proximal anastomosis to reduce aortic manipulation
- Using off-pump coronary artery bypass for those with severe atherosclerosis or deep hypothermic arrest for replacement of the ascending aorta

- Using cell-saver to process mediastinal blood
- Using post-pump arterial filters, using single aortic cross-clamping during CPB, or avoiding cross-clamping
- Providing adequate acid–base management
- Flooding the surgical field with carbon dioxide to evacuate air
- Controlling hyperglycemia, hypotension, and hyperthermia and managing pain
- Encouraging early mobility
- Providing rapid treatment of atrial fibrillation and anticoagulation
- Providing early intervention and treatment for cerebral ischemia

Stroke

Embolic stroke

Up to 6% of cardiac surgery patients experience a stroke as a complication, usually within the first 24–48 hours. Most stokes are ischemic. Manipulation of the ascending aorta is a primary risk factor for developing intraoperative or postoperative (most common) embolic strokes. Strokes are also often preceded by a period of atrial fibrillation (Afib), especially if Afib persists for extended periods (48 hours). Afib is treated with cardioversion or pharmacological rate control with anticoagulation.

Hemorrhagic strokes

However, hemorrhagic strokes may result from anticoagulation needed for cardiopulmonary bypass, causing a ruptured cerebral artery. This results in not only a lack of oxygen and nutrients but also edema that causes widespread pressure and damage. About 30% of infarcts may undergo hemorrhagic conversion. Multiple infarcts of varying sizes may occur following cardiac surgery. Serial computed tomography scans may be necessary for diagnosis as the initial scan may be negative. Diffusion weighted magnetic resonance imaging is most sensitive but may not be possible and may show preoperative undiagnosed infarcts.

Stroke risk factors

Risk factors for strokes associated with cardiac surgery are multiple and can include preexisting conditions, habits, and health problems as well as factors related to the surgical procedure. The most common etiology is cerebral microembolization, occurring during coronary artery bypass graft surgery. Risk factors include the following:
- Preexisting carotid disease (present in about 30%)
- Female gender
- Surgery involving manipulation of the aorta; calcified aorta
- Advanced age
- History of previous stroke
- Critical condition and weakened state before surgery
- Compromised ventricular function
- History of diabetes mellitus or renal failure
- History of unstable angina, recent myocardial infarction, hypertension, and low-cardiac output syndrome
- Peripheral vascular disease
- Pulmonary hypertension
- Development of postoperative atrial fibrillation (increases risk two to five times)
- History of smoking
- Prolonged cardiopulmonary bypass surgery
- Redo surgery

Stroke in patient

Stroke in the cardiac surgery patient is usually aimed at support in the early stage and prevention of secondary complications. Supportive treatments include the following:
- Provide oxygen support to maintain oxygen saturation at 92% or more

- Provide endotracheal intubation if necessary to maintain adequate ventilation
- Prevent hyperthermia as a 1°C–2°C increase in brain temperature can cause damage. Methods include antipyretics and cooling devices
- Monitor and maintain blood pressure (BP) at levels that allow for adequate perfusion. Hypertension should be controlled gradually, avoiding hypotension. In many cases, BP falls after a stroke without medications. Hypotension is treated with fluid boluses or vasopressor
- Maintain glycemic control; hypoglycemia may present with symptoms similar to a stroke, and hyperglycemia increases morbidity from strokes. Serum glucose should be maintained at 80–140 mg/dL
- Administer aspirin as it may improve outcomes, if not contraindicated

Strokes

Strokes most commonly occur in the right or left hemisphere, but the exact location and the extent of brain damage determine the presenting symptoms. If the frontal area of either side is involved, there tends to be memory and learning deficits. Some symptoms are common to specific areas and help to identify the area involved.

Right hemisphere

This results in left paralysis or paresis and a left visual field deficit that may cause spatial and perceptual disturbances so patients often have difficulty judging distance. Fine motor skills may be impacted, resulting in trouble dressing or handling tools. People may become impulsive and exhibit poor judgment, often denying impairment. Left-sided neglect (lack of perception of things on the left side) may occur. Depression, short-term memory loss, and difficulty following directions are common. Language skills usually remain intact.

Symptoms of strokes vary according to the area of the brain affected.

Left hemisphere

This results in right paralysis or paresis and a right visual field defect. Depression is common, and people often exhibit slow, cautious behavior, requiring repeated instruction and reinforcement for simple tasks. Short-term memory loss and difficulty learning new material or understanding generalizations are common. Difficulty with mathematics, reading, writing, and reasoning may occur. Aphasia (e.g., expressive, receptive, global) is common.

Brain stem

Because the brain stem controls respiration and cardiac function, a brain attack frequently causes death, but those who survive may have a number of problems, including respiratory and cardiac abnormalities. Strokes may involve motor or sensory impairment or both.

Cerebellum

This area controls balance and coordination. Strokes in the cerebellum are rare but may result in ataxia, nausea, vomiting, headaches, and vertigo.

Brachial plexus injury

Sternal retraction may result in brachial plexus injury, often associated with fracture of the first rib. Patients may complain of impaired sensation, including numbness, paresthesia, pain, and weakness related to T8–T1 injury, along the ulnar nerve distribution, often in the fourth and fifth fingers. Radial nerve deficits may also occur but are rare. Diagnosis is based on symptoms, electromyography results, motor–sensory conduction velocities, and somatosensory-evoked potentials. In most cases, no treatment is necessary as symptoms resolve over a few months, although a few patients may have persistent problems. Patients complaining of pain may get relief from amitriptyline, gabapentin, or carbamazepine.

Paraplegia

Paraplegia is a rare complication of aortic dissection and may also result from use of an intra-aortic balloon pump. With the coronary artery bypass graft procedure, paraplegia usually occurs following an episode of hypotension in patients with preexisting hypertension and vascular compromise.

Peripheral nerve assessment

Radial	The radial nerve branches from the brachial plexus and enervates the dorsal surface of the arm and hand, including the thumb and fingers two, three, and four. Sensation is evaluated by pricking the skin in the webbed area between the thumb and the index finger. Movement is evaluated by having the person extend the thumb, the wrist, and fingers at the metacarpal joint.
Ulnar	The ulnar nerve branches from the sciatic nerve and travels down the arm from the shoulder, traveling along the anterior forearm beside the ulna, to the palm of the hand. Sensation is evaluated by pricking the distal fat pad at the end of the small finger. Movement is evaluated by having the person extend and spread all the fingers.

Saphenous neuropathy

Saphenous neuropathy results from injury to branches of the saphenous nerve during harvesting of the saphenous vein. Indications include impaired sensation in the lower leg (medial aspect) and foot (to the great toe), especially if the vein is harvested distally to proximally. Endoscopic harvesting decreases the risk of saphenous neuropathy although it can still occur.

Radial neuropathy

Radial neuropathy is common, occurring in 42%–64% of patients during harvesting of the radial nerve. Indications include impaired sensation and paresthesias. Some patients may experience paralysis of vocal cords after cardiac surgery, especially with lengthy procedures. Indications include hoarseness and ineffective cough, putting the patients at risk for aspiration pneumonia. Most patients experience improvement in symptoms over a few months, but if symptoms persist, the injury may be permanent and surgical intervention (e.g., vocal cord medicalization, thyroplasty) may be indicated.

Post-pump hepatic failure

Hepatic dysfunction

Hepatic dysfunction is common after cardiac surgery, especially with prolonged cardiopulmonary bypass and multiple procedures. It is characterized by transient low-grade elevation of liver function tests. About a fourth of patients will develop hyperbilirubinemia and jaundice with bilirubin over 3 mg/dL, but less than 1% progress to post pump liver failure, which is characterized by coagulopathy, hypoglycemia, renal failure, encephalopathy, and refractory acidosis. Elevated bilirubin by itself is usually benign and self-limiting. Patients must be monitored carefully for coagulopathy during periods of hepatic dysfunction, as the impaired liver may not produce adequate clotting factors. Patients may exhibit jaundice or coagulopathy (i.e., a liver unable to produce sufficient clotting factors), hypoglycemia, renal failure, acidosis, or encephalopathy.

Treatment

Treatment includes the following:
- Coagulopathy: INR monitored and low doses of warfarin given, if anticoagulation is required

- Stress ulcers: proton pump inhibitor, such as pantoprazole, 40 mg intravenously or orally daily, for prophylaxis
- Hypoglycemia: Careful monitoring and administration of glucose
- Hyperammonemia/encephalopathy: Restrict protein; neomycin, 6 g; zinc sulfate, 600 mg daily; and lactulose, 30 mL four times daily with sorbitol
- Lactic acidosis: Sodium bicarbonate if base deficit over 10 mEq/L

Liver function studies

Bilirubin	Determines the ability of the liver to conjugate and excrete bilirubin: direct 0.0–0.3 mg/dL, total 0.0–0.9 mg/dL, and urine 0.
Total protein	Determines if the liver is producing protein in normal amounts: 7.0–7.5 g/dL Albumin: 4.0–5.5 g/dL Globulin: 1.7–3.3 mg/dL Serum protein electrophoresis is done to determine the ratio of proteins. Albumin/globulin (A/G) ratio: 1.5:1–2.5:1. (Albumin should be greater than globulin.)
Prothrombin time (PT)	100% or clot detection in 10–13 seconds. PT is increased with liver disease. INR (PT result/normal average): INR is less than 2 for those not receiving anticoagulation and 2.0–3.0 for those receiving anticoagulation. Critical value: This is more than 3 in patients receiving anticoagulation therapy.
Alkaline phosphatase (ALP)	17–142 U/L in adults (Normal values of ALP vary with method.) Indicates biliary tract obstruction if there is no bone disease
Aspartate aminotransferase (AST) serum (SGOT)	10–40 U/L (AST increases in liver cell damage.)
Alanine aminotransferase (ALT) serum (SGPT)	5–35 U/L (ALT increases in liver cell damage.)
Gamma-glutamyltrans-ferease (GGT) serum (SGTP)	5–55 U/L females; 5–85 U/L males (GGT increases with alcohol abuse.)
Lactate dehydrogenase (LD)	100–200 U/L (LD increases with alcohol abuse.)
Serum ammonia	150–250 U/L (Serum ammonia increases in liver failure.)
Cholesterol	Increases with bile duct obstruction and decreases with parenchymal disease

Gastrointestinal complications

Gastrointestinal (GI) complications are rare following cardiac surgery, and most complications occur about a week after surgery. Risk factors for GI complications include prolonged mechanical ventilation, septic shock, and impaired renal function or complications. Those developing GI complications have an increased mortality rate (50%), so prevention is essential. Complications are commonly associated with splanchnic (visceral) hypoperfusion resulting from decreased cardiac output, with resulting vasoconstriction, hypoxia, and general hypoperfusion, leading to ischemia. Indications include decreased or absent bowel sounds, abdominal pain, abdominal distention, nausea, and vomiting. Other GI complications can include ileus, upper GI bleeding, hepatic failure, acute pancreatitis, and cholecystitis. Proton pump inhibitors are given to those with nasogastric tubes to reduce the incidence of bleeding.

Paralytic ileus
Paralytic ileus is a bowel obstruction resulting from impairment of neural innervation of the intestines, usually related to infection, electrolyte imbalance, or surgical manipulation. Symptoms include decreased or absent bowel sounds, abdominal pain, inability to defecate, seepage of liquid feces, abdominal distention, nausea, vomiting, electrolyte imbalance, and dehydration. Paralytic ileus may be present for several days after cardiac surgery and usually clears by taking nothing by mouth with nasogastric suctioning. Total parenteral nutrition should be initiated, and medications that interfere with motility (e.g., narcotics, calcium channel blockers, anticholinergics) should be discontinued when possible. Metabolic imbalances must be corrected.

Pseudo-obstructions
Pseudo-obstructions (acute and massive colonic dilatation) are treated with neostigmine, 2 mg intravenously, to decompress a distended colon rapidly. In persistent cases of colonic distention of 12 cm or more, decompressive colonoscopy or surgical intervention may be necessary.

Mesenteric ischemia
Mesenteric ischemia is a rare complication of cardiac surgery, usually identified 5–10 days postoperatively. Most occurrences are nonocclusive, usually associated with splanchnic (visceral) ischemia, especially in older patients with atherosclerosis and dehydration. An intra-aortic balloon pump may cause atherosclerotic embolism, heparin-induced thrombocytopenia, and mesenteric thrombosis. Indications include paralytic ileus or severe acute abdominal pain. Patients may exhibit absent bowel sounds, and elevated lactate. Other complications, such as sepsis, hemodynamic instability, and gastrointestinal bleeding, may be present as well, obscuring the diagnosis. Mortality rate is high (> 65%) without prompt identification and treatment. Papaverine, 0.7 mg/kg/hr, may be given for 5 days or less if the problem relates to vasoconstriction. Surgical exploration and bowel resection may be necessary with intestinal necrosis.

Pharyngeal dysfunction with dysphagia
Pharyngeal dysfunction with dysphagia occurs in 3% or fewer patients who undergo coronary artery bypass graft and increases the risk of aspiration, both silent and overt. Prolonged intubation increases the risk with about half of patients intubated for more than 48 hours experiencing dysphagia. Risk factors include advanced age, type 1 diabetes, renal impairment, chronic obstructive pulmonary disease, and a history or perioperative occurrence of stroke. The bedside swallowing test may help to identify overt aspiration. The patient is carefully observed while swallowing 50 mL of water. Indications of aspiration include a decrease in oxygen saturation per oximetry, coughing, or choking. Patients may require dietary modifications to reduce the risk of aspiration and referral to an occupational or speech therapist to improve swallowing. In severe

cases, a feeding tube may be required to ensure adequate nutrition.

Renal

Acute renal failure

Acute renal failure is abrupt and almost complete failure of kidney function with a decreased glomerular filtration rate (GFR), occurring over a period of hours or days. It most commonly occurs in hospitalized patients but may occur in others as well. The blood urea nitrogen increases, and nitrogenous wastes are retained (azotemia). There are three primary categories, related to cause:

- Prerenal disorders, such as myocardial infarction, heart failure, sepsis, anaphylaxis, and hemorrhage result in hypoperfusion of the kidney and decreased GFR
- Intrarenal disorders include burns, trauma, infection, transfusion reactions, and nephrotoxic agents that cause damage to glomeruli or kidney tubules, such as acute tubular necrosis. Burns and crush trauma injuries release myoglobin and hemoglobin from tissues, causing renal toxicity or ischemia. With transfusion reactions, hemolysis occurs, and the broken down hemoglobin concentrates and precipitates in tubules. Medications, such as nonsteroidal anti-inflammatory drugs and angiotensin-converting enzyme inhibitors, may interfere with kidney function and cause hypoperfusion and ischemia
- Postrenal disorders involve distal obstruction that increases pressure in tubules and decreases GFR

Nonoliguric renal failure

Nonoliguric renal failure occurs when the serum creatinine increases, but urinary output remains 400 mL/24 hr or more. This form of renal failure is most common after cardiac surgery and may occur in patients with a history of renal dysfunction or other risk factors. Renal damage is less pronounced than with oliguric failure, and mortality rate is relatively low (5%–10%). Treatment includes hemodynamic support and fluids as well as high-dose diuretics.

Oliguric renal failure

Oliguric renal failure occurs with an increase in serum creatinine and a decrease in urinary output to 0.3–0.5 mL/kg/hr or more, persisting for 12–24 hours (usually an indication of RIFLE [risk, injury, failure, loss, end stage] criteria, category 3). Mortality rates are about 50%. Treatment includes renal replacement therapy. Risk factors include low-cardiac output, infections, stroke, and respiratory failure.

Acute renal failure patterns

After cardiac surgery, three typical patterns of acute renal failure occur:

- Abbreviated: This results from a transient episode of renal ischemia, occurring during surgery. The serum creatinine increases postoperatively, peaking at day 4 and then decreases. Urinary output generally remains adequate
- Overt: This results from impairment of cardiac function and ischemia during surgery. Postoperatively, the serum creatinine level rises to a higher level and then decreases slowly to normal levels over 7–14 days
- Protracted: This results from a period of ischemia during surgery followed by increased serum creatinine, but as the creatinine begins to return to normal levels, another injury to the kidneys

occurs as the result of a complication, such as infection or hypoperfusion/hypotension, causing the creatinine to rise again

Tubular necrosis

Acute tubular necrosis (ATN) occurs when a hypoxic condition causes renal ischemia that damages tubular cells of the glomeruli so they are unable to filter the urine adequately, leading to acute renal failure. Causes include hypotension, hyperbilirubinemia, sepsis, surgery (especially cardiac or vascular), and birth complications. ATN may result from nephrotoxic injury related to obstruction or drugs, such as chemotherapy, acyclovir, and antibiotics, such as sulfonamides and streptomycin. Symptoms may be nonspecific initially and can include life-threatening complications.

Symptoms:
- Lethargy
- Nausea and vomiting
- Hypovolemia with low-cardiac output and generalized vasodilation
- Fluid and electrolyte imbalance, leading to hypertension, central nervous system abnormalities, metabolic acidosis, arrhythmias, edema, and congestive heart failure
- Uremia, leading to destruction of platelets and bleeding, neurological deficits, and disseminated intravascular coagulopathy
- Infections, including pericarditis and sepsis
- Urinary sediment: tubular epithelial or granular (brown)

Treatment:
- Identifying and treating underlying cause and discontinuing nephrotoxic agents
- Supportive care
- Loop diuretics, such as furosemide (Lasix), in some cases

- Antibiotics for infection (e.g., pericarditis, sepsis)

Urinalysis

Color	Pale yellow/amber, which darkens when urine is concentrated or when blood or bile are present
Appearance	Clear but may be slightly cloudy
Odor	Slight; a foul smell with a bacterial infection, depending upon the organism; some foods, such as asparagus
Specific gravity	1.015–1.025; may increase if protein levels increase or if there is fever, vomiting, or dehydration
pH	Usually ranges between 4.5–8 with an average of 5–6
Sediment	Red cell casts from acute infections, broad casts from kidney disorders, and white cell casts from pyelonephritis; leukocytes $10/mm^3$ or more are present with urinary tract infections
Glucose, ketones, protein, blood, bilirubin, and nitrate	Negative; increase in urine glucose with infection (with normal blood glucose); frank blood from some parasites and diseases but also drugs, smoking, excessive exercise, and menstrual fluids; increased red blood cells from lower urinary tract infections
Urobilinogen	0.1–1.0 mg/dL

Renal function studies

Specific gravity	1.015-1.025; determines kidney's ability to concentrate urinary solutes
Osmolality (urine)	350–900 mOsm/kg/24 hr; shows early defects if kidney's ability to concentrate urine is impaired
Osmolality (serum)	275–295 mOsm/kg
Uric acid	Males: 4.4–7.6 mg/dL; females: 2.3–6.6 mg/dL; increased levels with renal failure
Creatinine clearance (24-hour)	Males: 85–125 mL/min/1.73 m^2; females: 75–115 mL/min/1.73 m^2 Evaluates the amount of blood cleared of creatinine in 1 minute; approximates the glomerular filtration rate
Serum creatinine	0.6–1.2 mg/dL; increases with impaired renal function, urinary tract obstruction, and nephritis; stable with normal functioning
Urine creatinine	Males: 14–26 mg/kg/24 hr; females: 11–20 mg/kg/24 hr
Blood urea nitrogen (BUN)	7–8 mg/dL (8–20 mg/dL > age 60); increases with impaired renal function, as urea is end product of protein metabolism
BUN/creatinine ratio	10:1; increases with hypovolemia; normal ratio with intrinsic kidney disease, though BUN and creatinine levels are increased

Loop diuretics

Diuretics increase renal perfusion and filtration, thereby reducing preload and decreasing peripheral and pulmonary edema, hypertension, congestive heart failure, diabetes insipidus, and osteoporosis. There are different types of diuretics: loop, thiazide, and potassium sparing.

Loop diuretics inhibit the reabsorption of sodium and chloride (primarily) in the ascending loop of Henle. They also cause increased secretion of other electrolytes, such as calcium, magnesium, and potassium. This can result in imbalances that cause dysrhythmias. Other side effects include frequent urination, postural hypotension, increased blood sugar, and increased uric acid levels. They are short-acting so are less effective than other diuretics for control of hypertension:

- Bumetanide (Bumex) is given intravenously after surgery to reduce preload or orally to treat heart failure
- Ethacrynic acid (Edecrin) is given intravenously after surgery to reduce preload
- Furosemide (Lasix) is used to control congestive heart failure as well as renal insufficiency. It is used after surgery to decrease preload and to reduce the inflammatory response caused by cardiopulmonary bypass (postperfusion syndrome)

Thiazide diuretics

Thiazide diuretics inhibit the reabsorption of sodium and chloride primarily in the early distal tubules, forcing more sodium and water to be excreted. Thiazide diuretics increase the secretion of potassium and bicarbonate, so they are often given with supplementary potassium or in combination with potassium-sparing diuretics. Thiazide diuretics are the first line of drugs for treatment of hypertension. They have a long duration of action (12–72 hours, depending on the drug) so they are able to maintain control of hypertension better than short-acting drugs. They may be given daily or 3–5 days a week. There are numerous thiazide diuretics, including:

- Chlorothiazide (Diuril)
- Bendroflumethiazide (Naturetin)
- Chlorthalidone (Hygroton)
- Trichlormethiazide (Naqua)

Side effects include dizziness, lightheadedness, postural hypotension, headache, blurred vision, and itching, especially during initial treatment. Thiazide diuretics cause sensitivity to sun exposure, so people should be counseled to use sunscreen.

Potassium-sparing diuretics

Potassium-sparing diuretics inhibit the reabsorption of sodium in the late distal tubule and collecting duct. They are weaker than thiazide or loop diuretics but do not cause a reduction in potassium levels; however, if used alone, they may cause an increase in potassium, which can cause weakness, irregular pulse, and cardiac arrest. Because potassium-sparing diuretics are less effective alone, they are often given in a combined form with a thiazide diuretic (usually chlorothiazide), which mitigates the potassium imbalance. Typical side effects include dehydration, blurred vision, nausea insomnia, and nasal congestion, especially in the first few days of treatment:

- Spironolactone (Aldactone) is a synthetic steroid diuretic that increases the secretion of both water and sodium and is used to treat congestive heart failure. It may be given orally or intravenously
- Eplerenone (Inspra) is similar to spironolactone but has fewer side effects so it may be used with patients who cannot tolerate the other drug

RIFLE

The RIFLE criteria for classifying renal failure helps to identify acute kidney injury and progressive renal dysfunction after cardiac surgery. RIFLE classifications include:

- Risk (most common) includes increased serum creatinine by 150% or decreased glomerular filtration rate (GFR) by 25% or more with urinary output of 0.5 mL/kg/hr or more over 6 hours
- Injury includes increased serum creatinine by 200% or decreased GFR by 50% or more with urine output of 0.5 mL/kg/hr or less over 12 hours
- Failure includes increased serum creatinine by 300%, decreased GFR by 75%, or serum creatinine 4 mg/dL or more or an acute rise in serum creatinine of 0.5 mg/dL or more with urine output 0.3 mL/kg/hr or less over 24 hours
- Loss is acute renal failure persisting 4 weeks or more
- End-stage kidney disease occurs after 3 months

Hemodialysis

Hemodialysis can be used intermittently to manage hyperkalemia, fluid overload, acid–base imbalances, and hypercatabolic state in patients at risk for renal failure. Blood flow through the dialysis cartridge is 300–500 mL/min. It may also be initiated with signs of uremia. Intermittent hemodialysis is contraindicated for patients who are hemodynamically unstable but should be done before signs of renal failure and a marked increase in creatinine, if possible. Temporary intermittent hemodialysis is performed by insertion of a catheter into the internal jugular or subclavian vein. The femoral vein is usually avoided except for short-term dialysis because of the risk of thrombosis. Treatments are usually done three times weekly for 3–4 hours. If patients are at risk for bleeding, heparin-free hemodialysis should be performed. If the patient requires long-term hemodialysis, then a fistula should be considered. Peritoneal dialysis is rarely used because it causes abdominal distention and glucose absorption and can result in respiratory compromise and peritonitis.

Continuous renal replacement therapy

Continuous renal replacement therapy circulates the blood by hydrostatic pressure through a semipermeable membrane. It is used in critical care and can be instituted quickly.

CVVH
Continuous venovenous hemofiltration (CVVH) pumps blood through a double-lumen venous catheter to a hemofilter, which

returns the blood to the patient in the same catheter. Blood flow rate is 250 mL/min. It provides continuous slow removal of fluid, is better tolerated with unstable patients, and does not require arterial access. It provides slow correction of electrolyte imbalances. CVVH has a lower risk of clotting than slow continuous ultrafiltration (SCUF). CVVH can be carried out in hypotensive or unstable patients with use of a blood pump. Electrolytes must be monitored carefully and replacement solutions provided as needed because so much fluid is removed.

CVVHD

Continuous venovenous hemodiafiltration (CVVHD) is similar to CVVH but uses a dialysate to increase clearance of uremic toxins. CVVHD is more effective for severe electrolyte imbalance or hypercatabolic state. Blood flow rate is 150–300 mL/min. CVVHD has a lower risk of clotting than SCUF.

SCUF

Slow continuous ultrafiltration (SCUF) has a blood flow rate of 50–80 mL/min. It filters but provides no replacement fluid; however, it can provide a negative fluid balance of 7 L or less. There is an increased risk of clotting because of the slow filtration rate, and SCUF is ineffective for hyperkalemia or uremia.

CAVH

Continuous arteriovenous hemofiltration (CAVH) circulates blood from an artery (usually the femoral artery) to a hemofilter, using only arterial pressure and not a blood pump. The filtered blood is then returned to the patient's venous system, often with added fluids to offset those lost. Only the fluid is filtered. CAVH is used during cardiac surgery to remove excess fluids before cardiopulmonary bypass is discontinued. However, its use postoperatively is limited because of the need for heparinization and the need for adequate arterial pressure necessary to achieve hemofiltration.

Oliguria

Oliguria may indicate acute kidney injury and should be treated aggressively to prevent further kidney damage. Measures include:
- Ensuring patency and correct positioning of a Foley catheter
- Maintaining optimal cardiac function by treating hypovolemia, controlling cardiac arrhythmias, improving contractility, and reducing increased afterload (allowing systolic blood pressure up to 150 mm Hg)
- Providing diuretics and other medications to increase output, including intravenous furosemide, chlorothiazide, or bumetanide. Furosemide may be given with dopamine and mannitol. If filling pressures are elevated, nesiritide is indicated. Hypertension may be treated with fenoldopam
- If the initial treatments are ineffective in improving output, then fluid intake may be limited and drug doses readjusted. Potassium supplements should be avoided. A diet high in essential amino acids is indicated, and renal replacement therapy may be needed

Electrolyte imbalances

Hyponatremia

Sodium regulates fluid volume, osmolality, acid–base balance, and activity in the muscles, nerves, and myocardium. It is the primary cation (positive ion) in extracellular fluid (ECF), necessary to maintain ECF levels that are needed for tissue perfusion (normal value: 135–145 mEq/L). Hyponatremia (< 135 mEq/L)

Hyponatremia may result from inadequate sodium intake or excess loss, through diarrhea, vomiting, or nasogastric suctioning. It can occur as the result of illness, such as severe burns, fever, syndrome of

- 70 -

inappropriate antidiuretic hormone, acute respiratory failure, and ketoacidosis. Medications that cause hyponatremia include thiazide diuretics and nonsteroidal anti-inflammatory drugs. In the postsurgical cardiac patient, hyponatremia is almost always associated with hyperglycemia. Hyponatremia may occur with severe heart failure and may develop with hypovolemia, normovolemia, or hypervolemia. Symptoms vary and include the following:

- Irritability to lethargy and alterations in consciousness
- Nausea and vomiting
- Generalized muscle weakness
- Cerebral edema with headache, seizures, and coma
- Dyspnea with Cheyne-Stokes respirations to respiratory failure

The underlying cause is identified and treated, and sodium replacement is provided.

Hypernatremia

Hypernatremia (> 145 mEq/L)
Hypernatremia may result from renal disease, diabetes insipidus, and fluid depletion. Hypernatremia is uncommon after cardiac surgery but is associated with hyperventilation and increases the risk of mortality to 40%–60%. It may also result from dehydration from fever, diarrhea, diabetes, or osmotic diuretics.
Symptoms include the following:

- Irritability to lethargy to confusion to coma
- Seizures and flushing
- Muscle weakness and spasms
- Thirst
- Disorientation
- Poor skin turgor and dry oral mucosa and tongue

Treatment includes identifying and treating the underlying cause, monitoring sodium levels carefully, and replacing intravenous fluids. With levels of 150 mEq/L, tromethamine is used to treat metabolic

acidosis rather than sodium bicarbonate, which may increase sodium levels more. A too rapid decrease in sodium levels may result in cerebral edema.

Hypokalemia

Potassium is the primary electrolyte in intracellular fluid (ICF) with about 98% inside cells and only 2% in extracellular fluid (ECF), although this small amount is important for neuromuscular activity. Potassium influences activity of the skeletal and cardiac muscles. Its level is dependent on adequate renal functioning because 80% is excreted through the kidneys and 20% through the bowels and sweat (normal values: 3.5–5.5 mEq/L).

Hypokalemia (< 3.5 mEq/L; critical value: < 2.5 mEq/L)

Hypokalemia is caused by a loss of potassium through diuresis after cardiac surgery and cardiopulmonary bypass, diarrhea, vomiting, gastric suction, diuresis, alkalosis, decreased potassium intake with starvation, nephritis, diuresis without adequate potassium replacement, insulin used to treat hyperglycemia, and metabolic/respiratory alkalosis. Symptoms include the following:

- Lethargy and weakness
- Paresthesias
- Dysrhythmias with abnormalities on the electrocardiograph: premature ventricular contractions, prolonged PR interval, ST-segment depression, and flattened T waves with U waves
- Muscle cramps with hyporeflexia
- Hypertension (with ventricular dysrhythmias) and hypotension
- Tetany

Hypokalemia is caused by a loss of potassium through diuresis after cardiac surgery and cardiopulmonary bypass, diarrhea, vomiting, gastric suction, diuresis, alkalosis, decreased potassium intake with starvation, nephritis, diuresis without adequate potassium replacement, insulin used to treat hyperglycemia, and metabolic/respiratory alkalosis.

The underlying cause is identified and treated, and potassium chloride is replaced by central line at 10–20 mEq/hr in a mix of 20 mEq potassium chloride in 0.45% normal saline. (Dextrose solutions may stimulate the production of insulin and lower potassium levels.)

Hyperkalemia

Hyperkalemia (> 5.5 mEq/L; critical value: > 6.5 mEq/L)

Hyperkalemia can result from high-potassium cardioplegic solutions, low cardiac output with oliguria, tissue ischemia, acute or chronic renal insufficiency, and medications (e.g., nonsteroidal anti-inflammatory drugs, angiotensin receptor blockers, β-blockers, angiotensin-converting enzyme inhibitors, potassium-sparing diuretics).

The primary symptoms relate to the effect on the cardiac muscle:
- Ventricular arrhythmias with increasing changes in the electrocardiogram, leading to cardiac and respiratory arrest
- Weakness with ascending paralysis and hyperreflexia
- Diarrhea
- Increasing confusion

Treatment includes identifying the underlying cause and discontinuing sources of increased potassium:
- Calcium gluconate (10 mL/10% solution over 2–3 minutes) to decrease cardiac effects
- Furosemide (20–40 mg intravenously [IV]) to increase potassium secretion
- Sodium bicarbonate shifts potassium into the cells temporarily

- Insulin (10 U regular IV in 50 mL 50% dextrose) and hypertonic dextrose shift potassium into the cells temporarily
- Albuterol (10–20 mg) per nebulizer to move potassium into cells
- Cation exchange resin (sodium polystyrene sulfonate [Kayexalate]) enema (50 g/150 mL water) every 2–4 hours to decrease potassium

Hypocalcemia

More than 99% of calcium is in the skeletal system with 1% in serum, but it is important for transmitting nerve impulses and regulating muscle contraction and relaxation, including the myocardium. Calcium activates enzymes that stimulate chemical reactions and has a role in coagulation of blood (normal values: 8.2–10.2 mg/dL).

Hypocalcemia (< 8.2 mg/dL; critical value: < 7 mg/dL)

Hypocalcemia may be caused by hypoparathyroidism and occurs after thyroid and parathyroid surgery, pancreatitis, renal failure, inadequate vitamin D, alkalosis, magnesium deficiency, and low serum albumin. After cardiac surgery, hypocalcemia may be caused by cardiopulmonary bypass, hemodilution, multiple transfusions of citrated blood products, low cardiac output, and sepsis.

Symptoms include the following:
- Tetany, tingling, seizures, and altered mental status
- Ventricular tachycardia
- Laryngeal spasm and inspiratory and expiratory wheezing
- Decreased myocardial contractility and cardiac output, hypotension, prolonged QT interval, bradycardic dysrhythmias, and muffled heart sounds

Tetany

Tetany is the most common manifestation of hypocalcemia and hypomagnesemia. It includes a range of neuromuscular symptoms related to spontaneous discharge in both the sensory and motor peripheral nerves. Muscle spasms and twitching may cause pain, and there may be sensations of tingling in the fingers and perioral area. Seizures may occur. Two signs are present with tetany.

Chvostek's sign
Chvostek's sign is elicited by tapping the muscles enervated by the facial nerves about 2 cm in front of the earlobe just inferior to the zygomatic arch. A positive response is twitching of the muscle. A positive response may also occur with respiratory alkalosis.

Trousseau's sign
Trousseau's sign is elicited by applying a blood pressure cuff to the upper arm and inflating it 20 mm Hg above systolic and leaving it in place for 5 minutes or less. A positive response occurs with increasing ischemia of the ulnar nerve: carpopedal spasm with the thumb adducted, the wrist and metacarpophalangeal joints flexed, and the interphalangeal joints extended with the

Hypercalcemia

Hypercalcemia (> 10.2 mg/dL; critical value :>12 mg/dL)

Hypercalcemia is not usually a complication of cardiac surgery but relates to increased intestinal or bone absorption or decreased calcium elimination. Hypercalcemia may be caused by acidosis, kidney disease, hyperparathyroidism, prolonged immobilization, and malignancies. Hypercalcemia may also result from some medications (e.g., thiazide diuretics, lithium carbonate) and acidosis. Crisis carries a 50% mortality rate. Symptoms include the following:

- Increasing muscle weakness with hypotonicity
- Anorexia, nausea, and vomiting
- Decreased renal function, polyuria, and polydipsia
- Constipation
- Bradycardia and cardiac arrest, shortened QT segments, depressed T waves, and heart block (e.g., first, second, third, bundle branch block)
- Altered mental status, psychosis, lethargy, and coma (if untreated)

The underlying cause is identified and treated, and loop diuretics, intravenous (IV) calcitonin, and IV fluids are given.

Hypophosphatemia

Phosphorus, or phosphate (PO_4), is necessary for neuromuscular and red blood cell function and the maintenance of acid–base balance; it also provides structure for teeth and bones. About 85% is in the bones, 14% in soft tissue, and 1% or less in extracellular fluid (normal values: 2.4–4.5 mEq/L). Hypophosphatemia(< 2.4 mEq/L; critical value:<1 mEq/L)

Hypophosphatemia occurs with severe protein–calorie malnutrition; excess antacids with magnesium, calcium, or albumin; hyperventilation; severe burns; and diabetic ketoacidosis. Most commonly, hypophosphatemia results from increased renal elimination of phosphorus related to respiratory alkalosis or stress related to surgery. Hypophosphatemia is often associated with hypomagnesemia and hypercalcemia. Symptoms include the following:
- Irritability, tremors, and seizures leading to coma
- Muscle pain, weakness, and tenderness
- Apprehension and anxiety
- Hemolytic anemia
- Decreased myocardial function, hypotension, and decreased stroke volume

- Respiratory depression and failure (Respiratory rate falls with rising phosphorus levels, but with respiratory alkalosis, respiratory rate increases)

The underlying cause is identified and treated, and phosphorus is replaced. Phosphorus infusion may result in rebound hyperphosphatemia, characterized by heart block or flaccid paralysis.

Hyperphosphatemia

Hyperphosphatemia (> 4.5 mEq/L; critical value: > 5 mEq/L)

Hyperphosphatemia occurs with renal failure, hypoparathyroidism, excessive intake, and neoplastic disease, diabetic ketoacidosis, muscle necrosis, and respiratory acidosis. Most cases relate to decreased renal function and glomerular filtration rate, 50 mL/min or less. At this point, the kidneys cannot effectively metabolize phosphorus. Respiratory acidosis results in rising carbon dioxide levels, which causes phosphorus to move from intracellular to extracellular fluid compartments. Metabolic acidosis (as in diabetic ketoacidosis) also leads to hyperphosphatemia. Symptoms can include the following:
- Tachycardia, hypotension, muffled heart sounds, prolonged QT interval, and pericardial friction rub
- Altered mental status
- Muscle cramping, hyperreflexia, paresthesia, and tetany
- Nausea and diarrhea

The underlying cause is identified and treated; hypocalcemia is corrected; normal saline intravenous fluids and antacids are provided; and emergent renal replacement therapy is given, if necessary.

Hypomagnesemia

Magnesium is the second most common intracellular electrolyte (after potassium); it activates many intracellular enzyme systems. Magnesium is important for carbohydrate and protein metabolism, neuromuscular function, and cardiovascular function (electrical conduction), producing vasodilation and directly affecting the peripheral arterial system. Hypomagnesemia is often associated with hypophosphatemia, hypocalcemia, and hypokalemia (normal values: 1.6–2.4 mEq/L).

Hypomagnesemia (< 1.6 mEq/L; critical value: < 1.2 mEq/L)

Hypomagnesemia occurs from hemodilution during cardiopulmonary bypass (CPB) but also occurs in an open-pump coronary artery graft procedure; it is also associated with low-cardiac output syndrome and prolonged mechanical ventilation. It is common in cardiac surgery patients, especially those undergoing CPB or diuretics.

Symptoms include the following:
- Neuromuscular excitability/tetany
- Confusion, headaches, dizziness, seizure, and coma
- Tachycardia with atrial and ventricular arrhythmias
- Respiratory depression
- Nonspecific changes in T waves, U waves, prolonged QT interval, widened QRS complex, and ST-segment depression (Peaked T waves and torsade de pointes may be evident.)
- Insulin resistance

The underlying cause is identified and treated, and magnesium replacement is provided with magnesium sulfate (2 g/100 mL solution) to raise the level to 2 mEq/L or more. The infusion is stopped if urinary output falls to less than 100 mL/4 hr.

Hypermagnesemia

Hypermagnesemia (> 2.4 mEq/L; critical value: > 4.9 mEq/L; fatal value: > 10 mEq/L)

Hypermagnesemia can occur with hypercarbia; it decreases respiratory muscle function and is associated with respiratory failure/ventilator dependence as well as renal failure or inadequate renal function, diabetic ketoacidosis, hypothyroidism, and Addison's disease. Symptoms include the following:

- Muscle weakness and lethargy
- Dilated pupils
- Seizures
- Decreased or absent bowel sounds
- Anorexia
- Hypotension and shallow respirations, and periods of apnea
- Ventricular dysrhythmias, bradycardia, or prolonged PR interval
- Complete heart block and cardiac arrest
- Dysphagia with decreased gag reflex
- Tachycardia with hypotension

The underlying cause is identified and treated; seizure precautions are taken; and infusion of insulin and glucose, calcium gluconate (10–20 mEq over 10 minutes) loop diuretics, fluid resuscitation, and dialysis are provided. If a patient develops severe respiratory depression, mechanical ventilation may be necessary. Some patients require a temporary pacemaker for marked bradycardia.

Nursing Interventions

Antidysrhythmics

Group 1A antidysrhythmics

Group 1A antidysrhythmics, such as quinidine, procainamide, and disopyramide, are sodium channel blockers, which alter the cell membranes of the myocardium, interfering with the autonomic nervous system control of pacemaker cells. Blocking sodium results in the following:

- Decreased automaticity of ectopic foci (abnormal sites of pacemaker activity)
- Increased refractory period
- Decreased conduction speed

Procainamide and disopyramide are most frequently used after cardiac surgery. Sodium channel blockers are used to treat atrial fibrillation, premature ventricular contractions, and ventricular tachycardia. Adverse effects include gastrointestinal upset (i.e., nausea, vomiting, diarrhea), hypotension, dizziness, confusion, tinnitus, delirium, fever, chills, thrombocytopenia, and dysrhythmias, and heart failure. Contraindications include complete atrioventricular block, conduction defects, and myasthenia gravis. Sodium channel blockers must be used with caution in patients with renal or hepatic impairment.

Procainamide
Procainamide (Pronestyl), a group 1A sodium channel blocker, is used primarily to treat life-threatening ventricular arrhythmias and to prevent atrial fibrillation and less frequently to convert, although its use has been supplanted by amiodarone. Other indications include suppression of premature atrial/ventricular complexes and treatment of Wolff-Parkinson-White syndrome.

Procainamide slows conduction, decreases systemic vascular resistance, and decreases cardiac conductivity. Dosage is 100 mg every 5 minutes to a maximum dosage of 1000 mg followed by a maintenance infusion of 2–4 mg/min to a therapeutic level of 4–10 µg/mL. The infusion rate should not exceed 25–50 mg/min. Adverse effects include nausea, hypotension, anorexia, hallucinations, psychosis, depression, fever, rash, and lupus syndrome.

Disopyramide
Disopyramide (Norpace), a group 1A sodium channel blocker, is used to:

- treat atrial and ventricular arrhythmias (especially lifae-threatening ventricular arrhythmias, paroxysmal supraventricular tachycardia) and Wolff-Parkinson-White syndrome
- treat and prevent atrioventricular reentry tachycardia and
- to prevent or convert atrial fibrillation

Disopyramide decreases the rate of diastolic depolarization, reduces automaticity, prolongs the refractory period of myocardial cells, and decreases the rate of the rise of the action potential. Dosage is 100–200 mg orally every 6 hours to a therapeutic level of 2–5 µg/mL. Adverse effects include torsades de points, ventricular tachyarrhythmias, urinary retention, constipation, nausea, dizziness insomnia, blurred vision, dry mouth, impotence, rash, itching, muscle weakness, heart failure, hypotension, and cardiac conduction disturbances.

Group 1B antidysrhythmics

Lidocaine
Lidocaine is a group IB antidysrhythmic that is used to manage acute ventricular arrhythmias associated with cardiac surgery or myocardial infarction. Lidocaine is also used as a local or infiltrating anesthetic. As an antidysrhythmic, lidocaine decreases diastolic depolarization, decreases automaticity of ventricular cells, and

increases the threshold of ventricular fibrillation. Dosage is 1 mg/kg intravenously initially followed by a maintenance infusion of 2–4 mg/min with a bolus of 0.5 mg/kg in 15 minutes or when the infusion rate is increased. The therapeutic level is 1–5 μg/mL. Lidocaine is contraindicated with heart failure, cardiogenic shock, second- or third-degree heart block, Stokes-Adams syndrome, and Wolff-Parkinson-White syndrome. Lidocaine should be used cautiously with hepatic or renal impairment. Adverse effects include dizziness, tremors, vision changes, seizures, cardiac arrhythmias, cardiac arrest, vasodilation and hypotension, nausea, vomiting, respiratory depression or arrest, and malignant hyperthermia.

Group IC antidysrhythmics

Propafenone
Group IC antidysrhythmics block sodium at the cell membrane, depressing automatic firing of the sinus node and slowing impulses to the atria, atrioventricular node, ventricles, and Purkinje fibers. They are used for ventricular arrhythmias, atrial fibrillation, and atrial flutter. Drugs include propafenone and flecainide . After cardiac surgery, propafenone can be used to slow ventricular response and convert to sinus rhythm. Adverse effects include headache, dizziness, dysrhythmias, tremor, visual disturbances, and exacerbation of heart failure. In some cases, propafenone may cause new dysrhythmias or worsen those that are preexisting. Propafenone is contraindicated with heart block and must be administered with care for those with heart failure, impaired hepatic function, and potassium imbalances. Potassium levels should be monitored routinely.

Group II antidysrhythmics

β-Adrenergic blockers (β-blockers)
Group II antidysrhythmics, β-adrenergic blockers (β-blockers), slow the heart rate, reduce hypertension, prevent dysrhythmias, and reverse ventricular remodeling, so they are classified as both antidysrhythmics and antihypertensives. β-Blockers block β_1 and β_2 receptors by competing with norepinephrine. Negative inotropic and chronotropic effects reduce blood pressure. They slow sinus node conduction and prolong conduction through the atrioventricular node, decreasing the ventricular rate, and improving contractility and cardiac output. They are effective in reducing tachycardia associated with exercises or stress because they block excessive sympathetic nervous stimulation at the sinus node. β-Blockers should not be used during decompensation and should be monitored carefully for those with airway disease, uncontrolled diabetes, slow irregular pulse, or heart block. Adverse effects include bradycardia, hypostatic hypotension, heart failure, hypoglycemia, nausea, vomiting, diarrhea, sleep disorders, and edema. Commonly used drugs after cardiac surgery include metoprolol (ventricular dysrhythmias), sotalol (ventricular tachycardia), esmolol (sinus tachycardia, supraventricular tachycardia, and postoperative hypertension), and labetalol (postoperative hypertension). Because β-blockers may precipitate heart block, pacemaker backup should be readily available during treatment with intravenous β-blockers.

β-blockers

Labetalol
Labetalol is a β-blocker with combined α_1-, β_1-, and β_2-blocking properties ($\beta:\alpha$ is 7:1 intravenous [IV] and 3:1 oral). The combination helps to prevent reflex tachycardia that can occur with some α-blocking drugs. Onset of action (IV) is within 10–15 minutes, but duration is 6 hours. Labetalol is especially indicated both pre- and postoperatively for aortic dissection. Dosage is 0.25 mg/kg bolus with follow-up doses of 0.5 mg/kg every 5 minutes (to a maximum of 300 mg) or a continuous infusion at 1–4 mg/min until blood pressure stabilizes.

Labetalol is contraindicated with sinus bradycardia, second- or third-degree heart block, heart failure, cardiogenic shock, or asthma and should be used cautiously with diabetes or hypoglycemia. Adverse effects include dizziness, vertigo, fatigue, heart failure, cardiac arrhythmias, peripheral vascular insufficiency, gastric pain, flatulence, constipation, nausea, vomiting, diarrhea, impotence, decreased libido, dyspnea, and cough. Labetalol may increase the risk of atrioventricular heart block if given concomitantly with calcium channel blockers.

Esmolol

Esmolol is a β_1 selective adrenergic blocker that decreases the sympathetic nervous system influence on the heart, reducing the heart's excitability and cardiac output. Esmolol blocks the release of renin and lowers blood pressure and heart rate. Onset of action is within 2 minutes; it peaks in 5 minutes, with a reversal in 10–20 minutes; thus, it is the preferred drug in the initial postoperative period for control of transient hypertension, although it is contraindicated with low-cardiac output. Dosage is initially 0.25 mg/kg or less to determine response and a repeat dose up to 5 mg/kg with a maintenance infusion of 50–100 µg/kg/min. As an antidysrhythmic, labetalol is used to treat sinus tachycardia and supraventricular dysrhythmias. Dosage is 500 µg/kg load followed by a maintenance infusion of 50–200 µg/kg/min. Both toxic and therapeutic effects are increased if labetalol is given concomitantly with verapamil. Adverse effects of labetalol include lightheadedness, midscapular pain, weakness, rigors, hypotension, bradycardia, urine retention, local inflammation, fever, and flushing.

Metoprolol

Metoprolol is a β_1 selective adrenergic blocker that decreases the sympathetic nervous system influence on the heart, reducing the heart's excitability and cardiac output. Esmolol blocks the release of renin and lowers blood pressure and heart rate. Metoprolol is commonly given to prevent

atrial fibrillation (Afib) [oral dose 25–100 mg twice daily] with an additional intravenous dose of 5 mg every 5 minutes for three doses if Afib occurs. Onset of action is within 2–3 minutes, peak in 20 minutes, and duration up to 5 hours. Metoprolol may be given long-term for treatment of angina pectoris (50 mg twice daily initially increasing to 200 mg or less twice daily as needed). Metoprolol is also sometimes used for early or late treatment of myocardial infarction. Metoprolol should be withheld if bradycardia is less than 45 bmp, heart block is present, or systolic pressure is less than 100 mm Hg. Adverse effects include laryngospasm, heart failure, cardiac arrhythmias, gastric pain, flatulence, constipation, nausea, vomiting, diarrhea, impotence, decreased libido, arthralgia, dyspnea, and bronchospasm.

Group III antidysrhythmics

Group III antidysrhythmics are potassium channel blockers that may be used to convert atrial fibrillation (Afib) to sinus rhythm

Amiodarone

Amiodarone (most effective) converts Afib and provides rate control. Amiodarone prolongs repolarization and the refractory period, increases the ventricular fibrillation threshold, and decreases peripheral resistance. Amiodarone is contraindicated with sinus node dysfunction, hypokalemia, and severe bradycardia. Adverse effects include hypotension (rapid infusion), pulmonary and hepatic toxicity, visual disturbances, heart failure, cardiac arrest, and cardiac arrhythmias.

Ibutilide

Ibutilide is effective for both Afib and atrial flutter. Adverse effects include ventricular arrhythmias, hypotension, hypertension, tachycardia, headache, and dizziness. It is contraindicated with quinidine, procainamide, amiodarone, and sotalol.

Dofetilide

Dofetilide selectively blocks potassium channels and may be used for those with contraindications to class I drugs because of left ventricular dysfunction or β-blockers because of bradycardia or chronic obstructive pulmonary disease. It is used to convert Afib or flutter to normal sinus rhythm and to maintain sinus rhythm. It is contraindicated with heart block and must be used cautiously with ventricular arrhythmias and renal or hepatic impairment. Adverse effects include headache, tingling in the arms, dizziness, nausea, diarrhea, ventricular arrhythmias, hypotension, and hypertension.

Group IV antidysrhythmics

Calcium channel blockers

Group IV antidysrhythmics, calcium channel blockers (CCBs), which can also be used as vasodilators, act as antidysrhythmics to prevent and treat supraventricular arrhythmias. CCBs block the flow of positive calcium ions into cells, relax smooth arterial muscles, decrease myocardial contraction, slow atrioventricular (AV) conduction, reduce heart rate, decrease coronary vascular resistance, dilate coronary arteries, and increase blood flow to coronary arteries, while reducing myocardial oxygen demand. Commonly used medications include the following:

- Verapamil (Calan): Used for supraventricular tachycardia; depresses myocardium and prolongs AV conduction time
- Diltiazem (Cardizem): Used to treat paroxysmal supraventricular tachycardia, AV node reentry tachycardia, and Wolf-Parkinson-White syndrome

Adverse effects include constipation (common), nausea, muscle cramps, orthostatic hypotension, bradycardia, heart block, myocardial infarction, headache, dyspnea, and hepatic toxicity. CCBs may exacerbate heart failure and should be avoided. CCBs should be used with caution with hypotension, marked bradycardia, aortic stenosis, severe left ventricular impairment, and liver or kidney disease. Patients with heart failure must be monitored carefully.

Antidysrhythmics classes

Antidysrhythmics include a number of drugs that act on the conduction system, the ventricles or the atria to control dysrhythmias. There are four classes of drugs that are used as well as some that are unclassified:

- Class I: three subtypes of sodium channel blockers (1A: quinidine procainamide, disopyramide; IB: lidocaine, mexiletine, phenytoin; IC: propafenone and flecainide)
- Class II: β-adrenergic blockers (esmolol, propranolol)
- Class III: slows repolarization (amiodarone, ibutilide, dofetilide, sotalol, dronedarone)
- Class IV: calcium channel blockers (diltiazem, verapamil)
- Unclassified: adenosine

Antidysrhythmic used

Atrial fibrillation or atrial flutter

Digoxin (Lanoxin) affects the conduction system and may cause bradycardia, heart block, nausea, vomiting, and central nervous system depression.

Diltiazem (Cardizem) affects the conduction system and may cause bradycardia, atrioventricular block, and decreased blood pressure (BP).

Ibutilide (Corvert) affects the conduction system and rarely has side effects.

Amiodarone (Cordarone) affects the atria and ventricles and may cause decreased BP and adverse hepatic effects.

Metoprolol (Lopressor) blocks β-adrenergic cardiac receptors, decreasing response to sympathetic nervous system. It may cause larynx-gospasm, heart failure, arrhythmias,

Antidysrhythmics

Paroxysmal supraventricular tachycardia	Adenosine Digoxin (Lanoxin) affects the conduction system and may cause bradycardia, heart block, nausea, vomiting, and central nervous system (CNS) depression. Verapamil (Calan) affects the conduction system and may cause decreased blood pressure, bradycardia, and heart failure.
Sinus tachycardia	Esmolol (Brevibloc)
Premature ventricular contractions	Lidocaine affects the ventricles and may cause CNS toxicity with nausea and vomiting. Procainamide (Pronestyl)
Ventricular tachycardia	Lidocaine Amiodarone (Cordarone) Procainamide
Ventricular fibrillation	Lidocaine
Atrial flutter	Digoxin Diltiazem (Cardizem) Ibutilide (Corvert) Verapamil Amiodarone Procainamide

peripheral vascular insuffi-ciency, hypotension, and pulmonary edema.

Carvedilol (Coreg) lowers BP and prevents reflex tachycardia seen with many other drugs. It is used to treat hypertension, heart failure, and left ven-tricular dysfunction after myocardial infarction. It may cause dizzy-ness, tinnitus, bradycardia, orthostatic hypertension, cardiac arrhythmias, pulmonary edema, and hypotension.

Sotalol (Betapace) blocks sympathetic response and decreases cardiac excitability, reducing cardiac output and oxygen consumption. It may cause heart failure, dizziness, tinnitus, disorientation, heart failure, cardiac arrhythmias, sinoatrial or atrioventricular nodal block, peripheral vascular insufficiency, pulmonary edema, and hypotension.

Magnesium sulfate has few adverse effects.

Supraventricular tachycardia
Adenosine affects the conduction system and may cause transient flushing, decreased blood pressure, and shortness of breath.

Diltiazem (Cardizem) affects the conduction system and may cause brady-cardia, atrioventricular block, and decreased blood pressure (BP).

Esmolol (Brevibloc) affects the con-duction system and may cause decreased BP, brady-cardia, and heart failure.

Propranolol (Inderal) affects the conduction system and may cause brady-cardia, heart block, and heart failure.

Procainamide (Pronestyl) affects the atria and ventricles and may cause decreased BP and electro-cardiographic abnormalities (widening of QRS and QT).

Vasodilators

Vasodilators may be used for arterial or venous dilation to improve cardiac function. These drugs may be used to treat pulmonary hypertension or generalized systemic hypertension. They may be used for patients who cannot tolerate angiotensin-converting enzyme inhibitors or angiotensin receptor blockers. Vasodilators may dilate arteries, veins, or both:

- Arterial dilation reduces afterload, improving cardiac output.
- Venous dilation reduces preload, reducing filling pressures.

Smooth muscle relaxants

Smooth muscle relaxants decrease peripheral vascular resistance but may cause hypotension and headaches.

Sodium nitroprusside (Nipride) dilates both arteries and veins. It is rapid in action and used for the reduction of hypertension and afterload in heart failure.

Nitroglycerin (Tridil) primarily dilates veins and is used intravenously to reduce preload for acute heart failure, unstable angina, and acute myocardial infarction. Nitroglycerin may also be used prophylactically after percutaneous coronary intervention to prevent vasospasm.

Hydralazine (Apresoline) dilates arteries and is given intermittently to reduce hypertension.

CCBs

Calcium channel blockers (CCBs) are primarily arterial vasodilators that may affect the peripheral and coronary arteries. General side effects include lethargy, flushing, abdominal and peripheral edema, and indigestion.

Dihydropyridine, such as nifedipine (Procardia), which should be avoided in older adults, and nicardipine (Cardene) are primarily arterial vasodilators, affecting both coronary and peripheral arteries, used to treat acute postoperative hypertension. Nicardipine may cause headache, nausea, vomiting, peripheral edema, and tachycardia. Clevidipine (Cleviplex) acts as a smooth muscle relaxant and arterial vasodilator, decreasing mean arterial pressure and systemic vascular resistance. Clevidipine is used postoperatively to treat hypertension without compromising cardiac function. Side effects are similar to nicardipine but can include atrial fibrillation and acute renal failure.

Benzothiazepine, such as diltiazem (Cardizem) and phenylalkylamine, such as verapamil (Calan), dilate primarily coronary arteries and are used for angina and supraventricular tachycardias.

ACEIS

Angiotensin-converting Enzyme Inhibitors (ACEIs) limit the production of the peripheral vasoconstricting angiotensin, resulting in vasodilation, which can cause a precipitous fall in blood pressure, so use must be carefully monitored. ACEIs result in decreased and increased cardiac output but usually do not affect heart rate. They are often the first line of drugs to be used for acute hypertension and heart failure and are used to prevent nephropathy in patients with diabetes. After surgery, ACEIs may be administered in the initial period for those with mild left ventricular dysfunction, even with mild-to-moderate renal impairment, although serum creatinine levels should be monitored. Hyperkalemia may occur with inhibition of aldosterone.

Captopril (Capoten) and enalapril (Vasotec) decrease afterload and preload for heart failure.

Enalapril promotes vasodilation and decreases systemic vascular resistance. Adverse effects include cough, hyperkalemia, and renal failure.

Enalapril
Enalapril (Vasotec) is an angiotensin-converting enzyme inhibitor with antihypertensive action, inhibiting the renin–angiotensin system and decreasing vasoactive substances that usually increase with cardiopulmonary bypass. Enalapril provides both venous and arterial vasodilation, reducing preload and afterload without

increasing heart rate. Onset of action for intravenous [IV] administration is 15 minutes with a peak in 1–4 hours and a duration of 6 hours. Oral medications have an onset of 1 hour, with a peak in 4–6 hours and a duration of 24 hours. Intravenous enalapril may be given for patients with impaired ventricular function and persistent hypertension if they are unable to take oral medications. Usual dose is 0.625–1.25 mg IV over 5 minutes every 6 hours (with a repeat dose after 1 hour if the response is inadequate, although peak action may be delayed for 4 hours in some patients). Adverse effects include headache, dizziness, fatigue, syncope, palpitations, hypotension (in sodium- or volume-depleted patients), nausea, vomiting, diarrhea, decreased hemoglobin and hematocrit, cough, and muscle cramps.

B-type natriuretic peptides

B-type natriuretic peptides (nesiritide [Natrecor]) A new type of vasodilator (noninotropic), which is a recombinant form of a peptide of the human brain. It decreases filling pressure and vascular resistance and increases urinary output but may cause hypotension, headache, bradycardia, and nausea. It is used short term for worsening decompensated congestive heart failure.

Selective specific dopamine D$_1$-receptor agonists

Selective specific dopamine D1-receptor agonists, such as fenoldopam (Corlopam) are peripheral dilators affecting renal and mesenteric arteries and can be used for patients with renal dysfunction or those at risk for renal insufficiency. Fenoldopam is a rapid-acting peripheral and renal vasodilator that can be used to treat postoperative hypertension and is useful in patients with renal insufficiency as it increases glomerular filtration rate, renal blood flow, and excretion of sodium. It may cause a reflex tachycardia and hypokalemia.

Fenoldopam is rarely used postoperatively to treat hypertension but is usually used to protect the kidneys during surgery or to control hypertension when an immediate response (within 5 minutes) is necessary. Small doses used for renoprotective purposes usually do not result in hypotension.

Hydralazine

Hydralazine is an antihypertensive and peripheral vasodilator that acts on smooth muscle to cause arterial vasodilation, decreasing peripheral resistance. Hydralazine helps to maintain or increase both renal and cerebral blood flow. Hydralazine is commonly used as needed to control blood pressure when pressure remains unstable after the patient is transitioned to oral medications. Dosage is usually 10 mg intravenously (IV) injected slowly over 1 minute or 20–40 mg intramuscularly every 15 minutes until blood pressure responds and then every 6 hours. Hydralazine is fairly rapid acting with onset at 5–10 minutes (peaking at 20 minutes). Adverse effects include headache, peripheral neuritis, palpitations, tachycardia, angina, anorexia, nausea, vomiting, diarrhea, rash, arthralgia, fever, and nasal congestion. Hydralazine increases the effects of β-blockers, so the dosage of a concomitant β-blocker may need to be adjusted. Oral medications should be given with food. Medication should be withdrawn slowly to prevent rebound hypertension. Patients may experience orthostatic hypotension, especially in the morning, during hot weather, and with exercise or ingestion of alcohol.

ARBS

α-adrenergic receptor blockers (ARBs) block α receptors in the arteries and veins, causing vasodilation but may cause orthostatic hypotension and edema from fluid retention. Blocking the angiotensin receptors results in decreased aldosterone, which can lead to increased renal sodium and water secretion.

ARBs are used to manage hypertension and are contraindicated in patients with bilateral renal artery stenosis. Commonly used medications include:

- Labetalol (Normodyne) is a combination peripheral α-blocker and cardiac β-blocker and is used to treat acute hypertension, acute stroke, and acute aortic dissection
- Phentolamine (Regitine) is a peripheral arterial dilator that reduces afterload and is used for pheochromocytoma

Vasopressors

Adrenergic agonists

Adrenergic agonists are vasopressors (vasoconstrictors) with effects similar to norepinephrine or epinephrine. Adrenergic agonists can bind directly to adrenergic receptors to promote the release of norepinephrine, block norepinephrine reuptake, or inhibit activation of norepinephrine. Adrenergic agonists are used to control hypotension in the cardiac surgery patient when the patient is unresponsive to other measures. Following cardiac surgery, about 40% of patients require vasopressor support and 20% inotropic support.

Two classifications of adrenergic agonists include the following:

- Catecholamines: Epinephrine, norepinephrine, dopamine, and dobutamine
- Noncatecholamines: Phenylephrine

Classification
Adrenergic agonists usually have specific actions or combined actions, depending on the particular agent, and the action may be dose dependent; thus, the same drug at different dosages may have different actions. Adrenergic agents are classified according to which receptors they stimulate and the resultant action:

- α_1: vasoconstriction
- α_2: inhibition of norepinephrine release and vasodilation
- β_1: increased heart rate, blood pressure, contractility, cardiac output, automaticity, and conduction velocity
- β_2: bronchodilation
- D_1: vasodilation
- D_2: inhibition of norepinephrine release and vasodilation
- V_1: increased pulmonary vascular resistance and vasoconstriction (capillaries/arterioles)

Phenylephrine

Phenylephrine, a selective α_1-adrenergic agonist, increases both systolic and diastolic blood pressure but has little effect on β receptors in the heart. It is used postoperatively to manage mild-to-moderate hypotension, especially for patients with a high cardiac index and marked vasodilation. It can treat vascular failure associated with shock or drug-induced hypotension/hypersensitivity. With phenylephrine, systemic vascular resistance usually increases while cardiac output decreases, and heart rate may increase or decrease. Dosage depends on the clinical picture but usually ranges from 2–200 mcg/min. Adverse effects can include hypoperfusion with resultant splanchnic and renal ischemia. Phenylephrine may increase myocardial oxygen consumption and worsen metabolic acidosis. Other adverse effects include necrosis with extravasation, decreased urine formation and dysuria, cardiac arrhythmias, nausea, vomiting, dizziness, headache, tremors, and central nervous system depression. Phenylephrine is contraindicated with monoamine oxidase inhibitors, severe hypertension, ventricular tachycardia, pulmonary edema, and narrow-angle glaucoma. Phenylephrine is used with caution in diabetics and asthmatics. Adequate fluid resuscitation should be given before administration of phenylephrine.

Epinephrine

Epinephrine stimulates α_1, β_1, and β_2 receptors and is used postoperatively primarily for inotropic effects to improve cardiac function and increase stroke volume, to control refractory hypotension, to increase heart rate, or to treat cardiac arrest. The effects on different receptors vary according to dosage:

- Low dose (< 0.2 mcg/kg/min): Stimulation of β_2 receptors results in bronchodilation and vasodilation
- Moderate dose (0.008–0.06 mcg/kg/min): Stimulation of β_1 receptors increases blood pressure, cardiac output, and contractility
- High dose (0.5–4.0 mcg/min): Stimulation of β_1 receptors (for a chronotropic effect) increases heart rate
- Highest dose (> 2 mcg/min): Stimulation of α_1 receptor results in vasoconstriction

Adverse effects relate to dosage with high dosages more likely to cause severe hypertension, myocardial ischemia, tachycardias, and tachyarrhythmias. Other adverse effects include hyperglycemia (sometimes requires insulin drip), metabolic acidosis (with serum bicarbonate levels, 17–21 mEq/L), especially if epinephrine is administered within 6–8 hours of surgery. Extravasation may result in tissue necrosis. Heart and glucose monitoring must be done continuously.

Norepinephrine

Norepinephrine stimulates α_1 and β_1 receptors, resulting in both vasoconstriction and inotropic action. Norepinephrine also has some stimulation of β_1 receptors, resulting in bronchodilation. Norepinephrine is used postoperatively for severe hypotension when volume replacement is not adequate and may be given with fluid resuscitation. It is the most frequently used vasopressor to treat hypotension/shock associated with cardiopulmonary bypass. The dosage usually begins at 2–20 mcg/min with dosages titrated to reach optimal response (mean arterial pressure of at least 70 mm Hg). Adverse effects include increased myocardial oxygen consumption and workload, hyperglycemia, and metabolic acidosis. Reception of α_1 receptors may result in visceral ischemia and renal damage. High doses may cause vasoconstriction that impairs peripheral perfusion and can lead to necrosis, so peripheral pulses, capillary refill time, and skin temperature and color should be assessed frequently.

Vasopressin

Vasopressin is released in the body in response to cardiopulmonary bypass (CPB), sometimes resulting in post-CPB vasoconstriction, but the levels fall with prolonged hypotension; some people have low levels of vasopressin. Vasopressin is a potent vasoconstrictor that is used to treat vasodilatory shock after CPB when other measures (e.g., fluid resuscitation, inotropes, norepinephrine) are unsuccessful. Vasopressin may also be used for cardiac arrest associated with ventricular fibrillation or pulseless ventricular tachycardia and for milrinone-related hypotension. Vasopressin stimulates V_1 receptors and causes vasoconstriction of capillaries and small arterioles and increases secretion of corticotropin, which, in turn, stimulates the adrenal cortex to produce cortisol, helping to regulate blood pressure. Dosage varies from 0.01–0.1 U/min per intravenous infusion. Adverse effects relate to hypoperfusion and ischemia with end-organ damage, hyponatremia, and increased systemic vascular resistance. Vasopressin must be used very cautiously in patients with preexisting vascular disease.

Peripheral perfusion assessment

Assessment of peripheral perfusion can indicate venous or circulatory impairment.

Venous refill
Begin with the patient lying supine for a few moments, and then position the feet in a dependent position. Observe the veins on the dorsum of the foot, and count the seconds before normal filling. Venous occlusion is indicated with times of 20 seconds or more.

Capillary refill
Grasp the toenail bed between the thumb and index finger, and apply pressure for several seconds to cause blanching. Release the nail, and count the seconds until the nail regains normal color. Arterial occlusion is indicated with times of 2–3 seconds or more. Check both feet and more than one nail bed.

Skin temperature
Using the palm of the hand and fingers, gently palpate the skin, moving distally to proximally, comparing both legs. Circulatory impairment is indicated by decreased temperature (coolness) or a marked change from proximal to distal.

Inotropic agents

Inotropic agents increase cardiac output and improve contractility of the myocardium for heart failure. Intravenous inotropic agents may increase the risk of death but may be used when other drugs fail. Oral forms of these drugs are less effective than intravenous.

Dopamine
Dopamine stimulates $\alpha1$, $\alpha2$, and $\beta2$, D1, and D2 receptors although $\beta2$ stimulation is less than with other adrenergic drugs. Dopamine can be used for vasoconstriction or inotropic and chronotropic effects, depending on dosage:
- Low doses (< 8 mcg/kg/min) stimulate D1 and D2 receptors, resulting in inhibition of norepinephrine and vasodilation
- Doses of 0.5–3.0 mcg/kg/min result in renal vasodilation
- Doses of 4–10 mcg/kg/min stimulate $\beta1$ receptors, providing positive inotropic and chronotropic effects
- High doses of 10 mcg/kg/min or more stimulate $\alpha1$ receptors, providing vasoconstriction by stimulating endogenous norepinephrine

Dopamine is used to improve cardiac output, increase blood pressure and renal perfusion, and (at high doses) treat hypertension. Adverse effects include hypertension, chest pain, tachyarrhythmias, dyspnea, ventricular dysrhythmias, and gangrene. Dopamine is contraindicated with pulmonary hypertension and tachyarrhythmias.

Dobutamine
Dobutamine, a synthetic catecholamine that is primarily a $\beta1$ agonist but also has some stimulation of $\alpha1$ and $\beta2$ receptors. Dobutamine improves cardiac output, treats cardiac decompensation, lowers systemic vascular resistance and blood pressure, and increases heart rate, improving contractility. Dobutamine is indicated especially for patients who cannot tolerate vasodilators and have decreased cardiac output but high systemic vascular resistance or pulmonary vascular resistance. Patients with mitral valve replacement or high pulmonary pressures may have more benefit from dobutamine than dopamine. Dosage is usually 2–20 mcg/kg/in with rapid response. Adverse effects include increased systolic blood pressure and heart rate as well as premature ventricular contractions (5%), hypotension, and local reactions. Dobutamine should be avoided with hypovolemia.

Phosphodiesterase III inhibitors

Milrinone (Primacor) Milrinone (preferred drug) increases the strength of contractions and causes vasodilation, decreasing systemic vascular resistance and pulmonary vascular resistance, especially indicated for patients with right ventricular failure. Other actions include increased cardiac output/cardiac index and stroke volume and decreased pulmonary artery occlusion pressure. Milrinone improves myocardial oxygenation. Milrinone usually has minimal effects on the heart rate. The initial dose is 50–75 mcg/kg with a maintenance infusion of 0.25–0.75 mcg/kg/min. Adverse effects include ventricular arrhythmias, hypotension, and headaches. Patients may need an adrenergic agonist to counteract pronounced vasodilation and replacement of potassium and magnesium to prevent dysrhythmias. Hypotension may occur during treatment, so patients must be monitored closely.

Inamrinone (Inocor) Inamrinone acts as a venous and arterial vasodilator and has hemodynamic effects that are similar to milrinone. The initial loading dose is 50–75 mg/kg over 2–3 minutes followed by a maintenance infusion of 10–30 mg/kg/min (total dose not to exceed 10 mg/kg/d) or repeat loading doses. Adverse effects include thrombocytopenia, nephrogenic diabetes mellitus, impaired liver function, and exacerbation of dysrhythmias.

Fluid Volume Management

Digitalis use

Digitalis, an inotrope most commonly administered in the form of digoxin (Lanoxin), is derived from the foxglove plant and is used to increase myocardial contractility and left ventricular output and slow conduction through the atrioventricular (AV) node, decreasing rapid heart rates and promoting diuresis. Digoxin does not affect mortality but increases tolerance to activity and reduces hospitalizations for heart failure. Therapeutic levels (0.5–2.0 ng/mL) should be maintained to avoid digitalis toxicity, which can occur even if digoxin levels are within the therapeutic range, so observation of symptoms is critical. Potassium imbalance may cause toxicity.

Toxicity

Symptoms of Toxicity	Treatment
Early signs Increasing fatigue, lethargy, depression, nausea, and vomiting Sudden change in heart rhythm, such as regular or irregular rhythm, and palpitations Sinoatrial or AV block, new ventricular dysrhythmias, and tachycardia (atrial, junctional, ventricular) Bradycardia	Discontinue medication. Monitor serum levels and symptoms. Digoxin immune Fab (Digibind) may be used to bind to digoxin and inactivate it if necessary. **Note:** A number of drugs, including amiodarone, may increase digoxin levels.

Methylene blue

Methylene blue inhibits nitric oxide, which is released in the body after cardiopulmonary bypass. Nitric acid can cause severe vasoplegia with marked peripheral vasodilation and hypotension associated with normal- or high-cardiac output, low central venous pressure, pulmonary artery occlusion pressure, and lower pulmonary vascular resistance. Methylene blue is used to treat vasodilatory shock although it is not approved by the Food and Drug Administration for this purpose. Methylene blue is also used to treat type III protamine reaction that results in catastrophic pulmonary vasoconstriction, cyanide poisoning, and drug-induced methemoglobinemia. Usual dosage for vasodilatory shock is 1–2 mg/kg intravenously over 20 minutes. Adverse effects include hypertension, temporary (about 10 minutes) low oxygen saturation, hypotension, dizziness, headache, nausea, vomiting, diarrhea, and abdominal pain. Patients must be carefully monitored for hypertension, urine discoloration, oxygen saturation, and methemoglobin levels and may need to have a reduced rate of norepinephrine infusion. Methylene blue should be used cautiously in those with glucose-6-phosphate dehydrogenase deficiency, anemias, and renal impairment.

Fluid balance/fluid deficit

Body fluid is primarily intracellular fluid (ICF) or extracellular fluid (ECF). By 3 years of age, the fluid balance has stabilized and remains the same throughout adulthood.
- ECF: 20%–30% (interstitial fluid, plasma, transcellular fluid)
- ICF: 40%–50% (fluid within the cells)

The fluid compartments are separated by semipermeable membranes that allow fluid and solutes (i.e., electrolytes, other substances) to move by osmosis. Fluid also moves through diffusion, filtration, and active transport. In fluid volume deficit, fluid is out of balance, and ECF is depleted; an overload occurs with an increased concentration of sodium and retention of fluid. Signs of a fluid deficit include the following:
- Thirsty
- Restless to lethargic
- Increased pulse rate and tachycardia
- Depressed fontanelles (infants)
- Decreased urinary output
- Normal blood, pressure progressing to hypotension
- Dry mucous membranes
- A 3%–10% decrease in body weight

Hypovolemia/fluid volume deficit

Hypovolemia/fluid volume deficit occurs when the loss of extracellular fluid is greater than the intake of fluid. Fluid and electrolytes are lost in equal proportions so serum electrolyte levels usually remain within a normal range unless there are other complications. Fluid volume deficit is classified by percentage of total body weight lost:
- Mild: 2%.
- Moderate: 2%–5%
- Severe: 8% or more

Hypovolemia is characterized by increased heart rate and arterial hypotension and decreased pulmonary arterial wedge pressure, central venous pressure, capillary refill time, and urinary output; there is also increased osmolality, specific gravity, hemoglobin, hematocrit, and blood urea nitrogen, and a serum creatinine ratio of over 30:1. Hypotension (postural or prolonged) and tachycardia are common. Hypovolemia may result from a net loss of blood during surgery, surgical hypothermia (resulting in vasodilation as the body warms), and intravenous fluid loss into interstitial spaces because of increased permeability of capillary beds. Hypovolemia is the most common cause of decreased cardiac output in the postsurgical period. Treatment includes fluid replacement, usually initially crystalloid and then colloid. Packed red blood cells may be required for hemodilution.

Discuss fluid/blood replacement

Estimating loss of fluids
Patients may have preexisting fluid deficit (e.g., from presurgical fasting) as well as fluid maintenance requirements. Estimating loss of fluids is done by multiplying the normal maintenance rate (calculated according to weight) by the number of hours of fasting:
- 10 kg or less: 4 mL/kg/hr
- 11–20 kg: additional 2 mL/kg/hr
- 21 kg or more: additional 1 mL/kg/hr

Surgical wound fluid losses (e.g., blood loss) or "third-space" losses must also be estimated, and fluids added to compensate. Surgeries are usually classified, according to the degree of trauma and expected fluid loss from redistribution, evaporation, and blood loss:

- Minimal (e.g., hernia repair): 2–4 mL/kg/hr
- Moderate (e.g., cholecystectomy): 4–6 mL/kg/hr
- Severe (e.g., colectomy): 6–8 mL/kg/hr

Additionally, fluids may need to be added in conditions in which there is excessive fluid loss preoperatively, such as from severe diarrhea, ascites, or fever. Blood loss should be estimated, based on suctioned blood and saturated dressings:
- 4 x 4 = 10 mL/blood
- Laparotomy pad = 100–150 mL/blood

Fluid shifts

Fluid shifts between spaces are controlled by differences in hydrostatic and colloid osmotic pressure (COP). While water usually moves freely among intracellular, intravascular, and interstitial spaces, sodium moves freely only between the intravascular and interstitial spaces and does not move passively into the intracellular spaces unless serum osmolality and sodium concentration decrease, pulling fluid into the intracellular space. Cardiac surgery results in decreased COP by increasing capillary permeability, shifting fluid from intravascular to interstitial spaces. Cardiopulmonary bypass (CPB) results in a 20%–30% increase in extracellular volume and increased sodium retention and potassium excretion. Each hour of CPB results in 800 mL fluid buildup; a 50% decrease is COP. Low levels of serum sodium postoperatively usually indicate total body fluid overload. Increased pulmonary capillary wedge pressure or decreased serum albumin pressures shifts fluid from the intravascular space to the interstitial space, resulting in pulmonary and tissue edema. Extracellular fluid (intravascular serum and interstitial fluid) is more easily lost than intracellular fluid. Electrolyte values reflect plasma levels and indicate the status of extracellular fluid.

Postoperative fluid management

Postoperative fluid management after cardiac surgery presents numerous challenges. Cardiopulmonary bypass (CPB) results in total body fluid and sodium overload, causing increased weight; this is not reflected in cardiac filling pressures because of capillary leak, decreased plasma and colloid osmotic pressure, and impaired myocardial function. Despite fluid overload, low-filling pressures are common with hypovolemia. Fluid administration is usually indicated to maintain intravascular volumes and adequate hemodynamics. Blood products and colloids are more effective in expanding intravascular volume than hypotonic solutions or crystalloids. If patients are well oxygenated, up to 1 L of crystalloid may be administered, followed by colloids if the response is not adequate. Colloids may include 5% albumin, which has less effect on coagulation than hydroxyethyl starches. Colloids with 5% albumin may increase interstitial fluid and cause decreased intracellular fluid. Hypertonic 25% albumin solutions reduce the amount of fluid necessary. Hydroxyethyl starch preparations are excellent volume expanders but may have adverse affects on renal function. Hypertonic saline solutions (3%) can increase intravascular volume but may cause hypernatremia.

Diuretics for fluid management

Diuretics are usually avoided for the first 6 postoperative hours, but once the patient has stabilized, diuretics may be used to excrete the sodium and fluid overload caused by cardiopulmonary bypass. Loop diuretics, such as furosemide, are the diuretics of choice for fluid management. Loop diuretics inhibit reabsorption of sodium and tubular water and may also improve the glomerular filtration rate (GFR). The usual dose for those with adequate renal function is 10–20 mg intravenously (IV); this dose can be repeated in 4 hours, although one dose may be sufficient for some patients. If hemodynamic status is unstable, an initial bolus of 40 mg may be followed by an infusion of 0.1–0.5 mg/hg/hr. If patients have developed tolerance to diuretics, a thiazide, such as chlorothiazide, 500 mg IV, may be given in conjunction with furosemide. Dopamine, 2–3 µg/kg/min, will also increase GFR and renal blood flow and may reduce the need for diuretics in patients with normal kidney function.

Intravenous fluid warmers

Intravenous fluid (IV) warmers warm fluids to body temperature to avoid inducing or worsening hypothermia, especially in geriatric patients. In cases of severe hypothermia, warmed fluids (104°F–108°F) may be administered to raise core temperature. Also, medications are absorbed more effectively in warmed fluids. There are numerous types of fluid warmers. Simple warmers warm fluid in the tubing as the tubing passes through the warming device. Some units are disposable and battery powered, and some are approved for both blood and fluids. Some units require special tubing or equipment. All must be monitored carefully. Special heating chambers may heat a number of IV fluid bags at one time in a cabinet-type structure. Intraoperative warming of IV fluids may prevent anesthesia-associated hypothermia.

Fluid replacement

Crystalloid solutions
Both colloids and crystalloid solutions (or a combination) are used as intravenous fluid therapy during surgery. Crystalloids are solutions of inorganic small molecules, glucose, or saline, dissolved in water. There are many types of crystalloid solutions:

- Hypotonic solutions are maintenance solutions used to replace water loss. Dextrose in water (D5W) is commonly used when patients have a water deficit and for those with sodium restriction

- Hypertonic solutions are used for hyponatremia (3% saline) and severe hypovolemic shock (3%–7.5% saline)
- Isotonic solutions are replacement solutions for loss of water and electrolytes. Isotonic crystalloids, such as normal saline (0.9%), Ringer's lactate (contains potassium), and Plasma-Lyte (contains potassium) are most commonly used. Different solutions contain different electrolytes (e.g., sodium, chloride, potassium, calcium, lactate, magnesium), so monitoring electrolytes is essential

Crystalloids are effective in restoring fluid volume, but blood replacement requires 3:1 administration of crystalloids, while colloids are 1:1 replacement, and rapid crystalloid administration may result in tissue edema. Crystalloids are usually given as initial resuscitation fluid in emergencies. Glucose in some solutions may prevent ketosis and hypoglycemia.

Colloids
Colloids are solutions (usually isotonic saline but available with glucose and in hypertonic solutions) with dissolved high-molecular-weight (large) noncrystalline molecules and electrolytes. Colloids stay in the intravascular space more readily than crystalloids, so they are effective volume expanders. They are used primarily for fluid replacement with severe intravascular deficits, such as from hemorrhage and in conditions with severe hypoalbuminemia or where protein loss is probable, such as severe burns. Colloids are derived from plasma proteins or synthetic glucose polymers. Colloids obtained from plasma contain albumin (5% or 25% solutions) and plasma protein fractions (5%). Jehovah Witnesses may object to receiving these solutions. Colloids obtained from synthetic glucose contain hydroxyethyl starches and gelatin. Colloids have more safety concerns than crystalloids. Allergic reactions (including anaphylaxis) may be caused by dextran, hydroxyethyl, and (to a

- 89 -

lesser degree) albumin. Bleeding may also result from a reduction in platelet aggregation, factor VII, and von Willebrand factor and prolonged partial thromboplastin time, so colloids should be avoided in patients with coagulopathies.

Hypertonic saline solution

Hypertonic saline solution (HSS) has a sodium concentration higher than 0.9% (normal saline) and is used to reduce intracranial pressure/cerebral edema. Concentrations usually range from 2%–23.4%, but 3% solutions may be used with cardiac surgery patients to treat total body fluid overload. HSS draws fluid from the tissue through osmosis. As edema decreases, circulation improves. HSS also expands plasma, increasing cerebral perfusion pressure, and counteracts hyponatremia that can occur in the brain after injury, causing increased intracranial pressure. It is administered as follows:

- Peripheral lines: HSS 3% or less only
- Central lines: HSS 3% or more

HSS can be administered continuously at rates varying from 30–150 mL/hr. Rates must be carefully controlled. Fluid status must be monitored to prevent hypovolemia, which increases the risk of renal failure. Laboratory monitoring includes the following:

- Sodium (every 6 hours) is maintained at 145–155 mmol/L. Higher levels can cause heart, respiratory, and renal failure
- Serum osmolality (every 12 hours) is maintained at 320 mOsmol/L. Higher levels can cause renal failure

Mannitol

Mannitol is an osmotic diuretic that increases excretion of both sodium and water and reduces intracranial pressure and brain mass. Mannitol may also be used to shrink the cells of the blood–brain barrier to help other medications breach this barrier. Mannitol is administered by intravenous infusion. It may be used during cardiopulmonary bypass to control blood pressure. Additionally, mannitol, 500 mL of 20%, is given with furosemide, 1 g, and dopamine, 2–3 μg/kg/min, to produce diuresis within 6 hours of onset of oliguria. Fluid and electrolyte balances must be carefully monitored as well as intake, output, and body weight. Concentrations of 20%–25% require a filter. Crystals may form if the mannitol solution is too cold, and the mannitol container may require heating (in 80°C water) and shaking to dissolve crystals; the solution should be cooled to body temperature or less before administration. Mannitol cannot be administered in polyvinylchloride bags as precipitates form. Side effects include fluid and electrolyte imbalance, nausea, vomiting, hypotension, tachycardia, fever, and urticaria.

Blood products

Platelet concentrates

Platelets may be administered to bleeding patients if the platelet count is 100,000/mm^3 or less after cardiac surgery. Since cardiopulmonary bypass renders some platelets dysfunctional, platelets may be administered even with levels 100,000/mm^3 or more. In the nonbleeding patient, platelets may not be indicated until the count reaches 20,000–30,000/mm^3. One unit increases the platelet count by 5000–10,000/mm^3. Platelet concentrates pose a risk for sensitization reactions and infectious diseases. Platelet concentrate is stored at a higher temperature (20°C–24°C) than red blood cells. This contributes to bacterial growth, so it is more prone to bacterial contamination than other blood products. An increase in temperature within 6 hours should be considered an indication of possible sepsis. Platelets should be administered through a 170 μm filter. If a patient's hematocrit is 30% or less or the patient has hypofibrinogenemia, then platelet function will be impaired; the patient may need infusion of cryoprecipitate and red blood cells to increase hematocrit. Platelets may increase filling pressures, which will lower hematocrit and precipitate fluid overload.

Fresh frozen plasma

Fresh Frozen Plasma (FFP) (obtained from a unit of whole blood frozen 6 hours or less after collection) includes all clotting factors and plasma proteins, so each unit administered increases clotting factors by 2%–3%. FFP may be used for deficiencies of isolated factors, excess warfarin therapy, and liver disease–related coagulopathy. It may be used for patients who have received extensive blood transfusions but continue to hemorrhage. It is also helpful for those with antithrombin III deficiency. FFP should be warmed to 37°C before administration to avoid hypothermia. ABO compatibility should be observed if possible, but it is not required. Some patients may become sensitized to plasma proteins. FFP is usually not given during surgery unless partial thromboplastin time or prothrombin time is prolonged 1.5 times or more. Plasma, as with platelets, may increase filling pressures, lowering hematocrit and precipitating fluid overload.

Blood Products Commonly Used for Transfusions

Red blood cells	Red blood cells (RBCs) may be administered after cardiac surgery primarily to increase the oxygen-carrying function of blood to prevent ischemia. RBCs are usually administered when the hematocrit falls to 26% or less. Blood filters with pore sizes of 170 μm or more should be used with all transfusions, and blood lines should be flushed with isotonic solutions (usually normal saline). Lactated Ringer's solution and dextrose 5% in water may result in red cell hemolysis.
Fresh whole blood	Fresh whole blood (< 6 hours old) contains clotting factors and platelets and has a hematocrit of 35%, so it provides a balanced replacement. However, it is not available from many blood banks.
Recovered blood (cell-saver or hemo-filtration blood)	Cell-saver blood is captured, filtered, rinsed with heparinized saline, and reinfused. It does not contain clotting factors or platelets and may contain minimal amounts of heparin. Blood recovered by hemofiltration from the extracorporeal circuit does retain platelets and clotting factors, but this procedure is usually not recommended.
Packed red blood cells (PRBCs)	PRBCs should be warmed to 30°C or more (optimal 37°C) to prevent hypothermia and may be reconstituted in 50–100 mL of normal saline to facilitate administration. PRBCs are necessary if blood loss is about 30% (1500–2000 mL) [hemoglobin ≤ 7]. Above 30% blood loss, whole blood may be more effective. PRBCs are most frequently used for transfusions. One unit usually contains approximately 200 mL of red blood cells, 30 mL plasma, and 100 mL of Optisol AS. One unit will usually raise the hematocrit in a 70-kg patient by 3%. PRBCs contain no clotting factors, so if multiple units are administered, then fresh frozen plasma may also be necessary.
Auto-transfusion	Mediastinal blood is reinfused through 20–40 μm filters but not washed. This procedure is associated with an increased risk of infection; if more than 500 mL is reinfused, patients may experience coagulopathy with an elevated INR, a partial thromboplastin time, and D-dimers and decreased fibrinogen.

Cryoprecipitate

Cryoprecipitate is the precipitate that forms when fresh frozen plasma (FFP) is thawed. It contains fibrinogen (150–250 mg), factor VIII-C (80–100 U), von Willebrand factor (40%–50%), factor XIII, and fibronectin. One unit of FFP provides about 15 mL of cryoprecipitate, which is mixed with 15 mL plasma and pooled into 6 U of concentrate—about 200 mL. This component may be used to treat hemophilia A and hypofibrinogenemia. Cryoprecipitate may be used in patients who have recently had thrombolytic therapy. Usually 1 U is administered for every 7–10 kg. It should be administered through a 170 μm filter 4–6 hours after thawing. Formulas to calculate the required dose include:

- Blood volume = 70 mL/kg x weight in kilograms
- Plasma volume = blood volume x (1 – hematocrit)
- Required fibrinogen (mg): 0.01 x plasma volume x (target level – current level)
- Bags of required cryoprecipitate: target milligrams of fibrinogen (250 mg/bag)

Blood administration

Jehovah Witnesses

Jehovah Witnesses have traditionally shunned transfusions and blood products as part of their religious beliefs. In 2004, the *Watchtower,* a Jehovah Witness publication presented a guide for members. When medical care indicates the need for blood transfusion or blood products and the patient or family members are practicing Jehovah Witnesses, this may present a conflict. It is important to approach the patient or family with full information and reasons for the transfusion or blood components without being judgmental, allowing them to express their feelings. In fact, studies show that while adults often refuse transfusions for themselves, they frequently allow their children to receive blood products, so one should never assume that an individual would refuse blood products based on the religion alone. Jehovah Witnesses can receive fractionated blood cells, thus allowing hemoglobin-based blood substitutes. The following guidelines are provided to church members:

Basic Blood Standards for Jehovah Witnesses	
Not acceptable	Whole blood: red cells, white cells, platelets, and plasma
Acceptable	Fractions from red cells, white cells, platelets, and plasma

Transfusion-related complications

Because there are a number of transfusion-related complications, transfusions are given only when necessary.

Infection

Bacterial contamination of blood, especially platelets, can result in severe sepsis. A number of infective agents (e.g., viral, bacterial, parasitic) can be transmitted, although increased testing of blood has decreased rates of infection markedly. Infective agents include HIV, hepatitis B and C, human T-cell lymphotropic virus, cytomegalovirus, West Nile virus, malaria, Chagas' disease, and variant Creutzfeldt-Jacob disease (from contact with meat infected with mad cow disease).

Transfusion-related acute lung injury (TRALI)

This respiratory distress syndrome is increasingly common and occurs in 6 hours or less. The cause is believed to be antileukocytic (anti-human leukocyte antigen) antibodies in the transfusion. It is characterized by noncardiogenic pulmonary edema (high protein level) with severe dyspnea and arterial hypoxemia. Transfusion must be stopped immediately and the blood bank notified. TRALI may result in death but usually resolves in 12–48 hours with supportive care.

Graft vs. host disease

Lymphocytes cause an immune response in immunocompromised individuals.

Lymphocytes may be inactivated by irradiation, as leukocyte filters are not reliable.

Post-transfusion purpura
Platelet antibodies develop and destroy the patient's platelets, so the platelet count decreases about 1 week after transfusion.

Transfusion-related immunosuppression
Cell-mediated immunity is suppressed, so the patient is at increased risk of infection and, in cancer patients, transfusions may correlate with tumor recurrence. This condition relates to transfusions that include leukocytes. Red blood cells cause a less pronounced immunosuppression, suggesting a causative agent is in the plasma. Leukoreduction is becoming more common to reduce transmission of leukocyte-related viruses.

Hypothermia
This may occur if blood products are not heated. A body temperature decrease of 0.5°C–1°C increases oxygen consumption by four times.

Hemodynamic Monitoring

Hemodynamic monitoring

Hemodynamic monitoring is the monitoring of blood flow pressures. For effective postoperative cardiac functioning, the correct relationship between high and low pressures must be maintained. During surgery, catheters are placed; the most common sites are the left atrium, right atrium, pulmonary artery, or superior vena cava.

Central venous pressure

Central venous pressure (CVP), the pressure in the right atrium or vena cava, is used to assess function of the right ventricles, preload, and flow of venous blood to the heart. Normal pressure ranges from 2–6 mm Hg but may be elevated after surgery to 6–8 mm Hg. Incorrect catheter placement or malfunctioning can affect readings.

Increased CVP is related to overload of intravascular volume caused by decreased function, hypertrophy, or failure of the right ventricle; increased right ventricular afterload, tricuspid valve stenosis, regurgitation, or thrombus obstruction; or a shunt from the left ventricle to the right atrium. It can also be caused by arrhythmias or cardiac tamponade.

Decreased CVP is related to low intravascular volume, decreased preload, or vasodilation.

Central venous catheter

Central venous catheters (CVCs) are used for hemodynamic monitoring; obtaining blood samples; and administering blood, fluids, or medication. CVCs are usually secured with a suture or staple and covered with a protective dressing. CVCs must have heparin flushes to prevent thrombus formation. Placement of a CVC may result in a number of complications, so the catheter must be monitored carefully. Complications include the following:

- Pneumothorax (usually during initial catheter placement) or hemothorax
- Perforation of vessels near the catheter, arterial puncture, or superior vena cava puncture
- Air embolism from negative intrathoracic pressure
- Thrombus formation, thrombophlebitis, or emboli
- Perforation of the pericardium
- Hemorrhage or formation of a hematoma (most often associated with placement of a CVC in the jugular vein)
- Cardiac arrhythmias from contact with the endocardium during placement
- Extravasation of fluids
- Local inflammation

- Central line–associated bloodstream infections primarily related to Staphylococcus aureus or S. epidermidis

Oxygen saturation

Hemodynamic monitoring includes monitoring oxygen saturation levels, which must be maintained for proper cardiac function. Changes in the oxygen saturation levels can indicate complications in the postsurgical patient. The central venous catheter often has an oxygen sensor at the tip to monitor oxygen saturation in the right atrium. If the catheter tip is located near the renal veins, this can cause an increase in right atrial oxygen saturation and a decrease near the coronary sinus.

Increased oxygen saturation may result from the left atrial shunt to the right atrial shunt, abnormal pulmonary venous return, increased delivery of oxygen, or a decrease in oxygen extraction.

Decreased oxygen saturation may be related to low-cardiac output with an increase in oxygen extraction or a decrease in arterial oxygen saturation with normal differences in the atrial and ventricular oxygen saturation.

Mixed venous gases

Mixed venous gases (MVG), especially venous oxygen saturation (SvO_2), are monitored for indications of respiratory failure, reduced oxygenation, anemia, and changes in cardiac output. MVG refers to venous blood that has returned to the heart from the superior and inferior vena cava and the coronary sinus. A sample from the right atrium may reflect primarily blood from the superior vena cava, which usually has a lower saturation (70%) than blood from the inferior vena cava (80%) or the coronary sinus (56%). The blood in the right ventricle and pulmonary artery is completely "mixed," and the saturation averaged. MVG is usually measured by

sampling through a pulmonary artery catheter. Normal values include the following:
- $PvCO_2$: 41–51 mm Hg (partial pressure of carbon dioxide in venous blood)
- PvO_2: 35–49 mm Hg (partial pressure of oxygen in venous blood)
- SvO_2: 60%–80% (oxygen saturation in venous blood)

If there is a decrease in SvO_2, then the oxygenation is not sufficient for tissue needs.

Left atrial pressure

Left atrial pressure may be monitored in the postsurgical period by way of a catheter inserted during surgery into the left atrium from the right superior pulmonary vein or through the left atrial appendage. Oxygen saturation of blood in the left atrium should be 100%.

Normal values are 1–2 mm Hg higher than right atrial pressure (4–12 mm Hg). Pressures above 12–14 mm Hg postsurgically are cause for concern.

Increased pressure may indicate an increase in end-diastolic pressure of the left ventricle, a decrease in function, hypertrophy, heart failure, or an increase in left ventricular afterload. An increase may also indicate mitral valve stenosis, backflow, or thrombus obstruction, a significant right-to-left shunt, excessive intravascular volume, tachycardia with arrhythmias, or cardiac tamponade.

Decreased pressure may indicate a decrease in intravascular fluid or insufficient preload.

Pulmonary artery pressure

Pulmonary artery pressure (PAP) is measured by a pulmonary artery catheter that is usually fed through the right ventricle to the main pulmonary artery; it is measured with the patient in the supine position (45° elevation or less).

Normal values are 10–20 mg Hg (mean PAP: 15 mm Hg). Postoperative rates should be less than 25 mm Hg. PAP is usually about 25%–34% of the systemic blood pressure rate. Oxygen saturation is usually about 80%.

Increased pressure may indicate pulmonary obstruction or embolus, left-to-right shunt, left ventricular failure, pulmonary hypertension, mitral stenosis, pneumothorax, lung/alveolar hypoplasia, hyperviscosity of blood, or increased left atrial pressure.

Decreased pressure may indicate a decrease in intravascular volume or cardiac output or obstruction of pulmonary blood flow.

Pulmonary artery mean

Pulmonary artery mean (PAM) provides the average pressure in the pulmonary artery during one cardiac cycle as PAP increases with contraction of the right ventricle and then decreases until the next contraction (mean PAM: 15 mm Hg).

Pulmonary artery catheter

The pulmonary artery catheter (PAC) can provide information about cardiac output, cardiac index, and intracardiac pressures and allows for earlier identification of left ventricular (LV) function than a central venous pressure line, which is associated with longer intubation and increased morbidity.

Pulmonary artery systolic (PAS) pressure indicates pressure from the tricuspid valve to the mitral valve and provides a good indication of pulmonary artery pressures (PAP). PAS increases with pulmonary hypertension.

Pulmonary artery diastolic (PAD) pressure indicates pressure between the pulmonic and aortic valves and provides a good indication of LV function (if there is no obstruction). PAD is usually slightly higher than pulmonary artery occlusive pressure (PAOP) and

pulmonary artery wedge pressure (PAWP) [≤ 5 mm Hg].

PAOP and PAWP indicate pressure between the distal end of the PAC and the aortic valve when the PAC balloon is inflated, providing better information about LV function than PAD. It is used to assess LV preload. Normal values are 4–12 mm Hg. Increased pressure may indicate left ventricular failure, mitral insufficiency, or mitral stenosis. The balloon should be inflated slowly and left deflated after reading.

Aortic blood flow

Aortic blood flow is assessed with esophageal Doppler monitoring (EDM) for evaluation of hypoperfusion (hypovolemia or septic shock), major organ dysfunction (renal or liver failure), hypotension, heart failure, cardiogenic shock, ruptures within the heart, mitral regurgitation, or tamponade. EDM may be used before, during, or after cardiac surgery. An esophageal probe is inserted through the patient's mouth while the patient is sedated, and Doppler ultrasound technology is used to monitor both the function of the left ventricle and the patient's fluid status. The probe may be left in place if the patient can tolerate it, but the patient should be monitored carefully for mucosal irritation. EDM can show the flow time, peak velocity, and minute distance, while stroke volume and cardiac output are calculated. Normal ranges include the following:
- Corrected flow time: 330–360 msec

Peak velocities are listed below:
- 20 years: 90–120 cm/sec
- 40 years: 80–110 cm/sec
- 60 years: 60–90 cm/sec
- 80 years: 40–70 cm/sec

Intra-arterial blood pressure monitoring

Intra-arterial blood pressure monitoring is done for systolic, diastolic, and mean arterial pressure (MAP) for conditions that decrease cardiac output, tissue perfusion, or fluid volume. A catheter is inserted into an artery, such as the radial (most frequently used), dorsalis pedis, femoral, or axillary, percutaneously or through a cut-down. Before catheter insertion, collateral circulation must be assessed by Doppler or the Allen test (used for the hand). In the Allen test, both the radial and ulnar arteries are compressed, and the patient is asked to clench the hand repeatedly until it blanches; then one artery is released, and the tissue on that side should flush. Then the test is repeated again, releasing the other artery.

Mean arterial pressure

The MAP is most commonly used to evaluate perfusion as it shows pressure throughout the cardiac cycle. Systole is one-third and diastole two-thirds of the normal cardiac cycle. The MAP for a blood pressure of 120/60 mm Hg (normal range 70–100 mm Hg) is as follows:

- [(Diastole x 2) + (systole x 1)]/3 = MAP
- (60 x 2 = 120) + (120) = 240/3 = MAP of 80

Mean arterial pressure (MAP) is the average arterial blood pressure and can be calculated with the diastolic pressure (DP) and systolic pressure (SP).

- Normal values are: 70–100 mm Hg
- Formula: MAP = DP + SP – DP/3

Systemic vascular resistance (SVR) is the resistance to blood flow in all vessels except pulmonary vessels.

- Normal values are: 800–1200 dynes/cm^5
- Formula: SVR = MAP – central venous pressure/cardiac output x 80

Pulmonary vascular resistance (PVR) is the resistance in the pulmonary arteries and arterioles against which the right ventricle has to pump during contraction. It is the mean pressure in the pulmonary vascular bed divided by blood flow. If PVR increases, stroke volume decreases.

- Normal values are: 50–250 dynes/cm^5
- Formula: PVR = pulmonary artery pressure – pulmonary capillary wedge pressure/cardiac output x 80

Perfusion pressure

The perfusion pressure, measured by the mean arterial pressure (MAP) that is necessary, may vary with different conditions and circumstances.

Pulse pressure

The pulse pressure is the difference between systolic and diastolic pressures, and this can be an important indicator. For example, with a decrease in cardiac output, vasoconstriction takes place in the body's attempt to maintain the blood pressure. In this case, the MAP may remain unchanged, but the pulse pressure narrows. Necessary values for MAP include the following:

- More than 60 mm Hg to perfuse coronary arteries
- Approximately 70–90 mm Hg to perfuse the brain and other organs, such as the kidneys, and to maintain cardiac patients and decrease the workload of the left ventricle
- Approximately 90–110 mm Hg to increase cerebral perfusion after neurosurgical procedures, such as carotid endarterectomy

Patients should be assessed for changes in pulse pressure that may be precipitated by medications, such as diuretics that alter fluid volume.

Cardiac output

Cardiac output is the amount of blood pumped through the ventricles during a specified period. Normal cardiac output is about 5 L/min (normal values: 4–8 L/min) at rest for an adult. With exercise or stress, this volume may multiply three or four times with concomitant changes in the heart rate and stroke volume. The basic formulation for calculating cardiac output is the heart rate per minute multiplied by measurement of the stroke volume, which is the amount of blood pumped through the ventricles with each contraction. The stroke volume is controlled by preload, afterload, and contractility.

- Cardiac output = heart rate x stroke volume

The heart rate is controlled by the autonomic nervous system. Normally, if the heart rate decreases, stroke rate increases to compensate, but with cardiomyopathies, this may not occur, so bradycardia results in a sharp decline in cardiac output. Cardiac index evaluates the cardiac output in terms of the body surface area (BSA):

- Cardiac index = cardiac output/BSA
- The normal values are 2.2–4.0 L/min/m²

Cardiac output is the amount of blood pumped through the ventricles, usually calculated in liters per minute.

- Normal values at rest are: 4–8 L/min
- Formula: Cardiac output = stroke volume x heart rate

Cardiac index is the cardiac output divided by the body surface area (BSA). This is essentially a measure of cardiac output tailored to the individual, based on height and weight, measured in liters/min per square meter of BSA.

- Normal values are: 2.2–4.0 L/min/m².
- Formula: Cardiac index = cardiac output/BSA.

Stroke volume is the amount of blood pumped through the left ventricle with each contraction, minus any blood remaining inside the ventricle at the end of systole.

- Normal values are: 60–100 mL/beat (1 mL/kg/beat)

- Formula: Stroke volume = cardiac index in L/min) x (heart rate per minute) x (1000)

Preload

Preload refers to the amount of elasticity in the myocardium at the end of diastole when the ventricles are filled to their maximum volume and the stretch on the muscle fibers is the greatest. The preload value is based on the volume in the ventricles. The amount of preload (stretch) affects stroke volume because as stretch increases, the resultant contraction also increases (Frank-Starling Law). Preload may decrease because of dehydration, diuresis, or vasodilation. Preload may increase because of increased venous return, controlling fluid loss, transfusion, or intravenous fluids.

Afterload

Afterload refers to the amount of systemic vascular resistance to left ventricular ejection of blood and pulmonary vascular resistance to right ventricular ejection of blood. Determinants of afterload include the size and elasticity of the great vessels and the functioning of the pulmonic and aortic valves. Afterload increases with hypertension, stenotic valves, and vasoconstriction.

Noninvasive hemodynamic monitoring

Thoracic electrical bioimpedance monitoring
Thoracic electrical bioimpedance monitoring is a noninvasive method of monitoring hemodynamics (e.g., cardiac output, blood flow, contractility, pre- and after-load, pulmonary artery pressure). Electrodes placed on the thorax measure changes in electrical output associated with the volume of blood through the aorta and its velocity. The monitor to which the electrodes are attached converts the signals to waveforms. The heart rate is shown on an electrocardiogram (ECG) monitor. The equipment calculates the cardiac output

based on the heart rate and fluid volume. A typical bioimpedence monitor has four sets of bioimpedence electrodes and three ECG electrodes. Height, weight, and length of the thorax are entered into the machine. Two sets of bioimpedance electrodes are placed at the base on the neck bilaterally and then two sets on each side of the chest. The distance between the neck electrodes and the chest electrodes (on the same side) must be entered into the machine. ECG leads are placed where they consistently monitor the QRS signal; they may need to be moved to achieve this.

LCOS

Low–cardiac output syndrome (LCOS) is a common complication of cardiac surgery, especially aortic valve surgery. LCOS results in an imbalance between the supply of oxygen and body needs, leading to metabolic acidosis. LCOS incidence relates to left ventricular ejection fraction (LVEF):

- 6% with a LVEF of more than 40%
- 12% with a LVEF of 20%–40%
- 23% with a LVEF of less than 20%

Causes include left ventricular dysfunction resulting in a transient decrease in perfusion, cardiac arrest from cardioplegia and myocardial stunning, decreased preload, increased afterload, dysrhythmias, and myocardial infarction. Indications include a decrease in pulmonary venous oxygen saturation (< 70%) and mean arterial pressure, confusion/altered mental status, hypotension, narrow pulse pressure, poor peripheral perfusion, reduced or absent urinary output, and need for inotropic support for more than 30 minutes or intra-aortic balloon pump (IABP) therapy. Treatment depends on the underlying cause but can include fluids, vasopressors, and inotropic agents. Epinephrine, norepinephrine, dopamine, or dobutamine is indicated for ejection fractions 20% below baseline. Vasopressors include phenylephrine, vasopressin, or epinephrine.

Nitroprusside and IABP therapy are used for increased afterload.

Preload alterations management

Preload refers to the volume of blood returning to the right or left heart at diastole (end of filling) as measured by central venous pressure, which measures the right filling pressure and pulmonary artery occlusion pressure, which reflects the left ventricular (LV) end-diastolic pressure. Adequate preload is essential for tissue perfusion. A decrease in preload after surgery may result from excessive diuresis, hypothermia, vasodilation related to warming, fluid resuscitation (volume may leave the vasculature for the interstitium with capillary leak), bleeding, vasodilators, and decreased LV compliance. Fluid resuscitation is determined by the type of fluid loss and hematocrit and the presence of coagulopathies. Fluid resuscitation should aim for a mean arterial pressure of 70–80 mm Hg. With bleeding or coagulopathy, blood products and coagulation factors may be needed. If there is no bleeding, then crystalloids or colloid may increase preload to a pulmonary artery occlusion pressure of 18–20 mm Hg. Even with decreased preload, inotropic agents should be avoided.

Increased afterload and SVR

Alterations in systemic vascular resistance (SVR) may occur after surgery, as indicated by afterload. Right-sided afterload is reflected by pulmonary vascular resistance (PVR) and left-sided, by SVR. Left-sided afterload increase is of most concern. Systolic blood pressure has the most pronounced effect on SVR. Cardiac output improves with reduction in afterload, but SVR often increases to compensate for low cardiac output. About 60% of postsurgical patients exhibit hypertension, usually because of vasoconstriction, which may relate to an inflammatory response to cardiopulmonary bypass or metabolic acidosis. Other causes of increased afterload include hypovolemia, hypothermia, hypercarbia, volume overload, cardiogenic shock, anxiety, and pain. Treatment includes vasodilators (e.g., sodium nitroprusside, nitroglycerin, milrinone), which often require administration of fluids to balance the decrease in preload and maintain intravascular fluid volume. Blood pressure must be monitored frequently with nitroprusside as it may cause a precipitous drop. An intra-aortic balloon pump may be required in severe cases.

Stroke volume index

Stroke volume index is the stroke volume tailored to the individual.
- Normal values are: 33–47 mL/beat/m2
- Formula: Stroke volume index = stroke volume/BSA

Left ventricular stroke work index

Left ventricular stroke work index measures the contractility of the left ventricle.
- Normal values are: 45–75 g/M/m2/beat
- Formula: Left ventricular stroke work index = stroke volume index x (mean arterial pressure – pulmonary capillary wedge pressure) x 0.0136

Pulmonary capillary wedge pressure

Pulmonary capillary wedge pressure/pulmonary artery wedge pressure/pulmonary artery occlusion pressure is an indirect measurement of preload or filling pressure of the left ventricle.
- Normal values are: 8–12 mm Hg

Incision Assessment and Management

Wound healing

<u>Four primary phases</u>
Hemostasis begins within minutes of incision when platelets begin to seal off the vessels and secrete substances that cause vasoconstriction. Thrombin is produced to stimulate the clotting mechanism, forming a fibrin mesh.

Inflammation (lag or exudative) occurs over days 1–4 with erythema, edema, and pain as the blood vessels release plasma, neutrophils, and polymorphonucleocytes to begin phagocytosis to remove debris and prevent infection. Neutrophils begin to fill in the incisional space.

Proliferation/granulation (fibroblastic) occurs over days 5–20 when fibroblasts produce collagen to provide support, and granulation tissue starts to form. New capillaries form. Basophils migrate to the incision and multiply. Epithelization and contracture of the wound occur.

Maturation (differentiation, remodeling, plateau) occurs after day 21. The fibroblasts leave the wound, and the collagen tightens to reduce scarring. The tissue gains tensile strength. This stage can take up to 2 years, and the wound can break down easily again during this phase.

Incisional sites

Cardiac surgery may involve a number of incisional sites, and all sites must be evaluated carefully.

Mediastinum is the midsternal incision is used for both cardiopulmonary bypass (CPB) and some non-CPB procedures; it is usually is 6–10 inches long.

Mini-thoracotomy incisions are usually about 2 inches in length. Procedures that require robotics or port access may result in an opening in the left chest wall (coronary artery bypass) or right chest wall (mitral repair or replacement).

Minimally invasive procedures may result in a mini-right thoracotomy in the third intercostal space for aortic valve surgery or fourth intercostal space for mitral valve surgery. Aortic value surgery may require an upper hemisternotomy and mitral valve procedures, a lower hemisternotomy.

Radial artery conduit is the incision that is 2–4 inches in length.

For saphenous vein conduit in emergency situations, the incision may be 3–6 inches long, but for planned procedures, an endoscopic harvesting may result in two or three 1.5–2.5 cm incisions.

Incision wound complications

Risk factors
Before surgery:
- Diabetes, hyperglycemia
- Obesity
- Older adult
- Nutritional impairment and dehydration
- Respiratory disease (chronic obstructive pulmonary disease, emphysema)
- Anemia
- Immunosuppression
- Venous impairment
- Medications (steroids, chemotherapy)
- History of smoking

During surgery:
- Bilateral harvesting of internal mammary arteries
- Increased numbers of bypass grafts
- Blood transfusions
- Improper technique (surgical/sterile)
- Hypothermia

- Ischemia
- Myocardial edema

After surgery:
- Return to surgery
- More than 5 U of blood or autotransfusion of mediastinal blood
- Prolonged ventilation and prolonged cardiopulmonary resuscitation

Surgical site infections

Category I: Superficial incisional
Comparison of data requires that precise and standardized definitions be used for the descriptions of surgical site infections. The Centers for Disease Control (CDC)/National Nosocomial Infections Surveillance (NNIS) developed the CDC Definitions of Nosocomial Infections to be used in reporting to NNIS and the National Surveillance System for Healthcare Workers. The type of wound is classified according to these definitions, and then the Risk Index is applied to determine the severity of infection as well as rates of infection. Surgical site infections are identified by degree of infection among other criteria.

Superficial incisional infection occurs within 30 days of surgery and involves only skin and subcutaneous tissue of the incision; the patient has one of the following:
- Purulent drainage
- Organisms isolated from culture of wound fluid or tissue
- Localized signs of infection (The wound is deliberately opened by the physician, resulting in positive wound culture.)
- Diagnosis of superficial infection by surgeon or attending physician

Category 2: Deep incisional
The second category of the Centers for Disease Control/National Nosocomial Infections Surveillance surgical site infections may include those wounds that have both superficial and deep incisional characteristics.

- 100 -

Deep incisional infection occurs within 30 days of surgery if there is no implant or within 1 year if an implant is in place. Infection appears related to the surgery and involves deep soft tissues (fascial and muscle layers) of the incision. The patient has one of following:

- Purulent drainage from an incision but not from the organ/space component of the surgical site
- Spontaneous dehiscence of the wound or deliberately opened by surgeon when the patient has one of the following symptoms:
  - a. fever (38°C), localized pain, or localized tenderness, unless the wound culture is negative
  - b. Abscess or other evidence of deep incision infection found on direct examination, histopathology, or radiology
  - c. Diagnosis of a deep incisional infection by the surgeon or attending physician

Category III: Organ/ space infection
The third category of the Centers for Disease Control/National Nosocomial Infections Surveillance surgical site infection definitions comprises organ/space infection.

Organ/space infection occurs within 30 days of surgery if there is no implant or within 1 year if there is an implant in place. Infection appears related to surgery and involves any part of the body, excluding the skin incision, fascia, or muscle layers, that is opened or manipulated during the operative procedure. Specific sites are assigned to organ/space infection to identify further the location of the infection. The patient has one of the following:

- Purulent drainage from a drain that is placed through a stab wound into the organ/space
- Organisms isolated from an aseptically obtained culture of fluid or tissue in the organ/space

- An abscess or other evidence of infection involving the organ/space that is found on direct examination, during reoperation, or by histopathology or radiology
- Diagnosis of an organ/space infection by a surgeon or attending physician

Preventive preoperative measures
Preventive preoperative measures can reduce the incidence of postoperative infections with cardiac surgery. Measures may include:

- Identifying any infections present preoperatively and treating them before surgery
- Applying collagen-gentamicin topically to the area of incision, especially in high-risk patients, such as diabetics and the obese (body mass index > 25)
- Avoiding shaving or using electrical clippers immediately before surgery to remove excess hair that might interfere with the procedure
- Showering before surgery (within 12 hours) and using the antimicrobial chlorhexidine gluconate in a no-rinse application the evening before surgery and the morning of surgery
- Applying topical mupirocin ointment intranasally for 1 day before surgery and 4 days after surgery
- Providing antibiotic prophylaxis with cephalosporin alone or combined with a glycopeptide if there is a high incidence of methicillin-resistant Staphylococcus aureus, usually one dose before surgery and one after

Cardiac postoperative site infections

Superficial
Superficial wounds (type 1) are characterized by cellulitis, with local tenderness, erythema, and serous drainage. Small areas of wound breakdown may occur with some purulent discharge. Treatment includes local wound care and antibiotics (6 weeks). Surgical exploration may be indicated if multiple areas begin to break down, suggesting a deeper

infection. Wire removal or curettage of infected bone may be necessary.

Mediastinitis

Mediastinitis (type 3) is infection of the deep soft tissue (including muscle and fascia) with purulent discharge and dehiscence along with fever, chills, local tenderness, chest wall pain, and an unstable sternum. *Staphylococcus aureus* infections usually have a rapid onset, occurring within 10 days. Occult infections—common with diabetics—often have delayed symptoms with collections of purulent material but few systemic signs. The white blood cell count is almost always elevated. Treatment may include surgical exploration and antibiotics for 6 weeks. Wounds may be closed or left open. In some cases, sternotomy and vacuum-assisted closure may be indicated.

Sternal dehiscence

Sternal wounds (type 2) are most often associated with coagulase-negative Staphylococcus and Staphylococcus aureus and are classified into three categories:

- Bone is sterile and viable
- Sternal osteitis is present in the proximal two-thirds of the sternum with non-viable bone.
- Sternal osteitis is present in the distal third of the sternum with nonviable bone

There may be significant purulent discharge. Treatment varies and can include antibiotics, surgical debridement, rewiring, and surgical repair with flap. If dehiscence occurs without infection, the goal is to retain the sternum.

Leg graft site infection

Saphenous vein harvesting leads to infection in the affected leg in 10%–20% of patients, especially in those with peripheral vascular disease, diabetes, or obesity. Cellulitis with breakdown of the wound, purulent discharge, tissue necrosis, hematoma, and edema may occur. Minor infections are treated with antibiotics and drainage. Deeper infections may require surgical exploration, placing of a Blake drain, and antibiotic irrigations.

White blood cell count

White blood cell (WBC)[leukocyte] count is used as an indicator of bacterial and viral infections and leukemia.

Normal WBC count for adults:
- 4,800–10,000/mm^3

Acute infection:
- 10,000+/mm^3; 30,000/mm^3 indicative of severe infection

Viral infection:
- 4,000/mm^3 and below

White blood cell differential

The differential provides the percentage of each different type of leukocyte. An increase in the WBC count is usually related to an increase in one type of leukocyte, often immature neutrophils, known as bands; this increase is referred to as a "shift to the left," an indication of an infectious process.

Cells	Normal Values	Changes
Immature neutrophils (bands)	1%–3%	Increase with infection
Segmented neutrophils (segs)	50%–62%	Increase with acute, localized, or systemic bacterial infections
Eosinophils	0%–3%	Decrease with stress & acute infection
Basophils	0%–1%	Decrease during the acute stage of infection
Lymphocytes	25%–40%	Increase in some viral and bacterial infections
Monocytes	3%–7%	Increase during the recovery stage of acute infection

Severe infections

There are a number of terms used to refer to severe infections and often used interchangeably, but they are part of a continuum.

Bacteremia
Bacteremia is the presence of bacteria in the blood but without systemic infection.

Septicemia
Septicemia is a systemic infection caused by pathogens (usually bacteria or fungi) present in the blood.

SIRS
Systemic inflammatory response syndrome (SIRS), a generalized inflammatory response, affecting many organ systems, may be caused by infectious or noninfectious agents, such as trauma, burns, adrenal insufficiency, pulmonary embolism, and drug overdose. If an infectious agent is identified or suspected, SIRS is an aspect of sepsis. Infective agents include a wide range of bacteria and fungi, including Streptococcus pneumoniae and Staphylococcus aureus. SIRS includes two of the following:
- Elevated (> 38°C) or subnormal rectal temperature (< 36°C)

- Tachypnea or partial pressure of carbon dioxide less than 32 mm Hg
- Tachycardia
- Leukocytosis (> 12,000/mm³) or leukopenia (< 4000/mm³)

Infections can progress from bacteremia, septicemia, and systemic inflammatory response syndrome (SIRS) to the following:

Sepsis
Sepsis is the presence of infection either locally or systemically in which there is a generalized life-threatening inflammatory response (SIRS). It includes all the indications for SIRS as well as one of the following:
- Changes in mental status
- Hypoxemia (< 72 mm Hg) without pulmonary disease
- Elevation in plasma lactate
- Decreased urinary output of less than 5 mL/kg/wt for 1 hour or more

Severe sepsis
Severe sepsis includes both indications of SIRS and sepsis as well as indications of increasing organ dysfunction with inadequate perfusion or hypotension.

Septic shock
Septic shock is a progression from severe sepsis in which refractory hypotension occurs despite treatment. There may be indications of lactic acidosis.

Multiorgan dysfunction syndrome
Multiorgan dysfunction syndrome is the most common cause of sepsis-related death. Cardiac function becomes depressed; acute respiratory distress syndrome may develop; and renal failure may follow acute tubular necrosis or cortical necrosis.
Thrombocytopenia appears in about 30% of those affected and may result in disseminated intravascular coagulation. Liver damage and bowel necrosis may occur.

Septic shock

Septic shock is caused by toxins produced by bacteria and cytokines that the body produces in response to severe infection, resulting in a complex syndrome of disorders.

Symptoms are wide-ranging:
- Initial: hyper- or hypothermia, increased temperature (> 38ºC) with chills, tachycardia with increased pulse pressure, tachypnea, alterations in mental status (dullness), hypotension, hyperventilation with respiratory alkalosis (partial pressure of carbon dioxide ≤ 30 mm Hg), increased lactic acid, unstable blood pressure, and dehydration with increased urinary output
- Cardiovascular: myocardial depression and dysrhythmias
- Respiratory: acute respiratory distress syndrome
- Renal: acute renal failure with decreased urinary output and increased blood urea nitrogen
- Hepatic: jaundice and liver dysfunction with an increase in transaminase, alkaline phosphatase, and bilirubin
- Hematologic: mild or severe blood loss (from mucosal ulcerations), neutropenia or neutrophilia, decreased platelets, and disseminated intravascular coagulation
- Endocrine: hyperglycemia and hypoglycemia (rare)
- Skin: cellulitis, erysipelas, and fascitis, and acrocyanotic and necrotic peripheral lesions

Septic shock is most common in patients over 50 years of age and those who are immunocompromised. There is no specific test to confirm a diagnosis of septic shock, so diagnosis is based on clinical findings and tests that evaluate hematologic, infectious, and metabolic states: a complete blood count, disseminated intravascular coagulation panel, electrolytes, liver function tests, blood urea nitrogen, creatinine, blood glucose, arterial blood gases, urinalysis, electrocardiogram, radiographs, and cultures of blood and urine.

Treatment must be aggressive and includes the following:
- Oxygen and endotracheal intubation as necessary
- Intravenous (IV) access with two large bore catheters and a central venous line
- Rapid fluid administration of 0.5 L normal saline or isotonic crystalloid every 5–10 minutes as needed (to 4–6 L)
- Monitoring urinary output to an optimum of more than 30 mL/hr
- Inotropic agents (e.g., dopamine, dobutamine, norepinephrine) if no response to fluids or fluid overload
- Empiric IV antibiotic therapy (usually with two broad-spectrum antibiotics for both gram-positive and gram-negative bacteria) until cultures return at which point antibiotics may be changed
- Hemodynamic and laboratory monitoring
- Removing source of infection (abscess, catheter)

Postsurgical nosocomial infections

About 5%–10% of cardiopulmonary bypass patients develop nosocomial infections, usually related to respiratory infections, bacteremia from central lines, urinary infections, and surgical site infections. Most bacteremias and surgical site infections are caused by Staphylococcus aureus, while respiratory infections are caused by Gram-negative infections. Prophylactic antibiotics are provided within 1 hour (cephalosporins) or 2 hours (vancomycin) of surgery. Drainage should be routinely cultured. Nasal mupirocin should be given before surgery and up to 5 days postoperatively to prevent a Staphylococcus infection. Chlorhexidine gluconate (0.12%) oral rinse is also effective in reducing infection. Hyperglycemia must be aggressively controlled. Catheters, central lines, and ventilators should be discontinued as soon as possible. Prolonged (up to 6 weeks) treatment with antibiotics may be necessary for infections.

Pain Management

Pain pathophysiology

The pathophysiology of pain comprises four steps.

Transduction
Afferent nociceptor nerve endings respond to injury (i.e., mechanical, thermal, chemical) by releasing mediators (i.e., prostaglandin, serotonin, histamine, bradykinin, substance P). These mediators activate more nociceptors. The pain impulse occurs with an action potential that results from an exchange of sodium and potassium ions at the cell membranes.

Transmission
The mediators activate the action potential and send the pain impulse from the transduction site, to the spinal cord and brain stem, and then to the thalamus and the cortical areas of higher functioning.

Perception
Once the brain perceives pain, it elicits a number of responses. The reticular response causes autonomic and motor reactions (withdrawing from a painful stimuli). The somatosensory response identifies the type, intensity, and location of pain. The limbic response provides an emotional response to pain.

Modulation
Stimuli are enhanced or inhibited by the hypothalamus, pons, and somatosensory cortex, affecting the individual response to pain.

Pain phases

Anticipation	Patients may exhibit or overtly express anxiety about pain before cardiac surgery. Anxiety may increase the perception of pain, so patients should be provided education about what type of pain may occur and a plan for dealing with the pain. Patients with a history of substance abuse may also have concerns about addiction that must be addressed.
Presence	When pain actually occurs, strategies for managing pain can affect the patient's level of comfort and anxiety and impact recovery. Both pharmacological and nonpharmacological (e.g., massage, heat, cold, relaxation, music therapy) approaches to pain management may be used.
Aftermath	Complications may arise if pain was not managed well. Pain management should be assessed with the patient after intervention to determine if the pain management method achieved a satisfactory reduction in pain.

Pain types

There are two primary types of pain, nociceptive and neuropathic, although some people may have a combination.

Nociceptive (acute) pain
Nociceptive or acute pain is the normal nerve response to a painful stimulus. Trauma that results in nociceptive pain can cause severe inflammation and damage to nerve endings. Nociceptive pain usually correlates with the extent and type of injury; that is, the greater the injury, the greater the pain. It may be procedural pain (related to wound manipulation and dressing changes) or

surgical pain (related to cutting of tissue). It may also be continuous or cyclic, depending on the type of injury. Nociceptive pain is usually localized to the area of injury and resolves over time as healing takes place. Pain may be somatic, resulting from the stimulation of nerves in the skin, or visceral, from compression of abdominal/thoracic viscera. Nociceptive pain is often described as aching or throbbing, but it generally responds to analgesia. Uncontrolled, this type of pain can in time result in changes in the nervous system that lead to chronic neuropathic pain.

Neuropathic (chronic) pain

While nociceptive pain is acute, neuropathic pain is chronic. Neuropathic pain occurs when there is a primary lesion in the nervous system or a dysfunction related to damaged nerve fibers. Neuropathic pain may be associated with conditions, such as diabetes, cancer, or traumatic injury to the nervous system. This type of pain is common in chronic wounds and is more often described as burning, stabbing, electric, or shooting pains. Often the underlying pathology causing the pain is not reversible. Pain may be visceral (diffuse or cramping pain of internal organs) caused by injuries to internal organs. It is also often diffuse rather than localized. It may also be somatic pain, involving muscles, skin, bones, and joints. Neuropathic pain is often more difficult to assess than nociceptive pain because the damage may alter normal pain responses. Neuropathic pain often responds better to antidepressants and antiseizure medications than analgesics.

TEA

Thoracic epidural analgesia (TEA) provides more effective pain control after cardiac surgery than parenteral administration of opioids; it is associated with fewer pulmonary complications because the duration of mechanical ventilation is usually reduced and there are fewer cardiac dysrhythmias. Patients receiving TEA must be monitored carefully for weakness in the lower extremities as an epidural hematoma may develop at the insertion site because of heparinization. Additionally, respiratory depression may occur and delay extubation. Onset of respiratory depression is rapid with fentanyl and sufentanil and delayed with morphine; however, respiratory depression most often occurs with higher doses of drugs, such as 4 mg of morphine. Rarely, neurologic complications can occur as the result of hemorrhage or infection. Infections are uncommon, but the risk increases after 48 hours. Other adverse effects include pruritus, nausea, vomiting, and urinary retention.

Pain assessment

Pain scale

Pain is subjective and may be influenced by the individual's pain threshold (the smallest stimulus that produces the sensation of pain) and pain tolerance (the maximum degree of pain that a person can tolerate). The most common current pain assessment tool for preteens and adolescents is the 1–10 pain scale:

- 0 = no pain
- 1–2 = mild pain
- 3–5 = moderate pain
- 6–7 = severe pain
- 8–9 = very severe pain
- 10 = excruciating pain

However, there is more to pain assessment than a number on a scale. Assessment includes information about the onset, duration, and intensity. Identifying what triggers pain and what relieves it can be very useful when developing a plan for pain management. Patients may show very different behavior when they are in pain. Some may cry and moan with minor pain, and others may exhibit little difference in behavior when truly suffering. Thus, judging pain by behavior can lead to the wrong conclusions.

PAINAD

Patients with cognitive impairment or the inability to verbalize pain may not be able to indicate the degree of pain, even by using a face scale with pictures of smiling to crying faces. The Pain Assessment in Advanced Dementia (PAINAD) scale may be helpful, especially for those with Alzheimer's disease. Careful observation of nonverbal behavior can indicate that the patient is in pain.

Respirations
Patients often have rapid, labored breathing as pain increases with short periods of hyperventilation (Cheyne-Stokes respirations).

Vocalization
Patients may remain negative in speech or speak quietly and reluctantly. They may moan or groan. As pain increases, they may call out, moan and groan loudly, or cry.

Facial expression
Patients may appear sad or frightened and may frown or grimace, especially on activities that increase pain.

Body language
Patients may be tense, fidgeting, pacing, and as pain increases, may become rigid, clench fists, or lie in fetal position. They may become increasingly combative.

Consolability
Patients are less distractible or consolable with increased pain.

Adverse systemic effects of pain

The adverse systemic effects of pain can negatively affect many body systems.

Cardiovascular
Tachycardia and increased blood pressure are common responses to pain, causing increased cardiac output and systemic vascular resistance. In those with preexisting cardiovascular disease, such as compromised ventricular function, cardiac output may decrease. The increased myocardial need for oxygen may cause or worsen myocardial ischemia.

Respiratory
An increased need for oxygen causes an increase in minute ventilation during splinting because pain can compromise pulmonary function. If the chest wall movement is constrained, tidal volume falls, impairing the ability to cough and clear secretions. Bed rest further compromises ventilation.

Gastrointestinal
Sphincter tone increases and motility decreases, sometimes resulting in ileus. There may be increased secretion of gastric acids, which irritate the gastric lining and can cause ulcerations. Nausea, vomiting, and constipation may occur. Reflux may result in aspiration pneumonia. Abdominal distention may occur.

Urinary
Increased sphincter tone and decreased motility result in urinary retention.

Endocrine
Hormone levels are affected by pain. Catabolic hormones, such as catecholamine, cortisol, and glucagon, increase, and anabolic hormones, such as insulin and testosterone, decrease. Lipolysis increases along with carbohydrate intolerance. Sodium retention can occur because of increased antidiuretic hormone, aldosterone, angiotensin, and cortisol. This, in turn, causes fluid retention and a shift to extracellular space.

Hematologic
There may be reduced fibrinolysis, increased adhesiveness of platelets, and increased coagulation.

Immune
Leukocytosis and lymphopenia may occur, increasing the risk of infection.

Emotional

Patients may become depressed, anxious, or angry; have a depressed appetite, and become sleep-deprived. These responses are most common in patients with chronic pain, who usually do not have the typical systemic responses of patients with acute pain.

PCA

Patient-controlled analgesia (PCA) allows the patient to control the administration of pain medication by pressing a button on an intravenous delivery system with a computerized pump. The device is filled with opioid (as prescribed) and must be programmed correctly and checked regularly to ensure that it is functioning properly and that controls are set. Most devices can be set to deliver a continuous infusion of opioid as well as a patient-controlled bolus. Commonly used medications after cardiac surgery include morphine sulfate, 1 g bolus and 0.3 mg/hr infusion; fentanyl, 10 μg bolus and 1 μg/kg/hr infusion; and remifentanil, 0.25–0.5 μg/kg bolus and 0.5 μg/kg/hr infusion. Each element must be set:

- Bolus: determines the amount of medication received when the patient delivers a dose
- Lockout interval: time required between administrations of boluses
- Continuous infusion: rate at which opioid is delivered per hour for continuous analgesia
- Limit (usually set at 4 hours): total amount of opioid that can be delivered in the preset time limit.

Most effective pain control

Thoracotomy
Epidural analgesia with opioids or regional local anesthetics (recommended) Intravenous (IV), intramuscular (IM), subcutaneous (SC), oral (PO) opioids and nonsteroidal anti-inflammatory drugs (NSAIDs), often combined as NSAIDs may reduce the amount of opioid required and

decrease adverse effects. NSAIDs must be used judiciously because of the potential for adverse effects:

- Patient-controlled analgesia (PCA) with opioids
- Cold compresses
- Intrathecal opioids or local anesthetics
- Transcutaneous electrical nerve stimulation

Note: NSAIDs should be avoided if there is a risk of bleeding.

Coronary artery bypass graft
The most effective pain control for coronary artery bypass includes:

- IV opioids or NSAIDs (recommended), often combined
- IV, IM, SC, and PO opioids and NSAIDs. Oral medications include acetaminophen with oxycodone.
- Intrathecal opioids

Note: Epidural and regional local anesthetics are rarely used and NSAIDs should be avoided with a risk of bleeding or renal hypoperfusion.

Complementary and alternative therapies

Complementary and alternative therapies are used as well as conventional medical treatment and should be included if this is what the patient or family wants, empowering the family to take some control. Complementary therapies vary widely and most can easily be incorporated into the plan of care. The National Center for Complementary and Alternative Medicine recognizes the following:

- Medical systems may include homeopathic, naturopathic medicine, acupuncture, and Chinese herbal medications
- Mind–body medicine can include support groups, medication, music, art, or dance therapy
- Biologically based practices include the use of food, vitamins, or nutrition for healing

- Manipulative/body-based programs include massage or other types of manipulation, such as chiropractic treatment
- Energy therapies may be biofield therapies intended to affect the aura (energy field) that some believe surrounds all living things. These therapies include therapeutic touch and Reiki
- Bioelectromagnetic-based therapies use a variety of magnetic fields

Naloxone (Narcan)

The opioid antagonist, naloxone (Narcan), is similar in structure to agonists, but it displaces agonists at μ receptors (less so at κ or δ receptors). It reverses activity of both endogenous opioids, such as endorphins, and exogenous opioids, such as natural (morphine sulfate) and synthetic (meperidine) opioids, and narcotic antagonist analgesics, such as nalbuphine and butorphanol. It may also serve as an antagonist to the antihypertensive effect of clonidine. Naloxone is primarily used to treat known or suspected narcotic overdose or narcotic depression related to the use of narcotics during surgery. Respiratory depression caused by excessive narcotics during surgery usually resolves quickly with naloxone (1–2 minutes), and the duration is quite short (30–45 minutes) as the drug is rapidly redistributed; thus, repeated doses or a continuous drip may be needed. If opioid analgesia is abruptly reversed, sympathetic stimulation may occur with resultant tachycardia, hypertension, and pulmonary edema. Withdrawal symptoms may occur in those who are opioid dependent.

World Health Organization pain ladder

The World Health Organization provides a pain ladder as guidance for pain management. Medications are usually given every 3–4 hours around the clock to prevent breakthrough pain.

Level 1	Mild pain	Pain management usually begins with acetaminophen or aspirin followed by nonsteroidal anti-inflammatory drugs (NSAIDs) as well as adjuvant drugs. There are a number of different NSAIDs, and people may respond differently to the different drugs; thus, patients should be monitored carefully and medications changed when indicated.
Level 2	Mild-to-moderate pain	Aspirin or acetaminophen is given with codeine and adjuvants. Medications include hydrocodone, oxycodone, and tramadol.
Level 3	Moderate-to-severe pain	Opioid drugs (e.g., morphine, fentanyl, oxycodone) are given to control this pain. Some nonopioid drugs and adjuvant drugs may also be used.

Adjuvant drugs include antianxiety medications, anticholinergics, anticonvulsants, antiemetics, antipruritics, and corticosteroids.

Epicardial Pacing

Epicardial pacing wires placement

Epicardial pacing wires may be attached directly to the exterior atria, ventricles, or both at the conclusion of surgery for cardiopulmonary bypass or valve repair or for patients with a risk of atrioventricular (AV) block because of medications used to control atrial fibrillation. Cold cardioplegia may precipitate transient sinus node or AV node dysfunction. While some surgeons avoid placing epicardial pacing wires because of concerns about bleeding and cardiac tamponade on removal, recommendations include placing at least one ventricular pacing wire. A typical configuration for pacing wires is atrial pacing wires placed in a plastic disk that is sutured low on the right atrium. The two ventricular wires are attached over the right ventricular wall. Atrial pacing wires may be used to record atrial activity and, with a standard electrocardiogram, can help to distinguish atrial, junctional, and ventricular arrhythmias. Pacing wires can also be used therapeutically to increase the heart rate to about 90 bpm to achieve optimal hemodynamics.

Classifying pacemakers

Temporary pacing modes for code positions I, II, and III after cardiac surgery include:
- Asynchronous atrial pacing: AOO.
- Atrial demand pacing: AAI
- Ventricular demand pacing: VVI.
- Atrioventricular (AV) sequential pacing (ventricular demand): DVI.
- AV sequential pacing (biventricular): DDD

Asystole or pulseless electrical activity

Patients with epicardial pacing may develop pulseless electrical activity if ventricular fibrillation (VF) occurs; the pacer should be turned off briefly to check for VF if asystole occurs. If there is no VF, then the pacing wires should be connected and epicardial pacing initiated in the DDD mode/90 bpm. If the arrest was witnessed, then the wires should be connected before initiating cardiopulmonary resuscitation (CPR) [1 minute delay]. If pacing is not successful in reestablishing a pulse within a minute, then external CPR should begin. After resuscitation efforts have begun, transcutaneous pacing may be attempted. Medications include the following:
- Bradycardia: epinephrine, 1 mg intravenous (IV) bolus every 3–5 minutes or an infusion of 2–10 μg/min, OR vasopressin, 40 U IV. Atropine, 1 mg IV every 3–5 minutes (to a total of 0.4 mg/kg)

North American Society of Pacing and Electrophysiology and British Pacing & Electrophysiology Group Pacemaker Codes		
I Chambers paced	II Chambers sensed	Response to sensing
A = atrium	A = atrium	T = triggers pacing
V = ventricle	V = ventricle	I = inhibits pacing
D = dual	D = dual	D = dual function (both T and I)
S = single chamber	S = single chamber	O = none
O = none	O = none	

III Programmable functions/rate response	IV Antiarrhythmic functions
O = none	O = none
R = rate responsive	P = paced (antitachycardia)
P = simple programmable	S = shock
M = multiprogrammable	D = dual function (P and S)
C = communicating	

- Bradycardia nonresponsive to epicardial pacing: atropine, 0.5 mg IV initially with 0.5–1 mg every 3–5 minutes (total dose of 3 mg) and attempt transcutaneous pacing; other medications: epinephrine, 2–10 μg/min, and dopamine infusion, 2–10 μg/kg/min)

Atrial pacing

Atrial (AV) pacing provides the best support for hemodynamics. Additionally, biatrial pacing after surgery may reduce the incidence of atrial fibrillation. To initiate atrial pacing, both atrial electrodes are connected to the pacemaker machine and the modes set at AOO (most common) or AAI. Pulse amplitude is usually 10–20 mA in the asynchronous mode; the pulse rate is set faster than the underlying rate. Normal AV conduction is necessary for atrial pacing, and it is ineffective for atrial fibrillation (Afib) or flutter. Indications include the following:

- Sinus bradycardia is treated by increasing heart rate with settings higher than the underlying rate
- Premature ventricular contractions are suppressed with pacing faster than the sinus mechanism
- Premature atrial complexes or prevention of Afib is suppressed with dual atrial pacing
- Junctional rhythm is suppressed
- Overdrive of supraventricular tachycardias is accomplished by interrupting the circuit and converting to sinus rhythm

Atrial overdrive pacing

Atrial overdrive pacing at high rates (≤ 800 bpm) may be used to control supraventricular tachycardias, such as atrial flutter, paroxysmal atrial or atrioventricular junctional reentrant tachycardia, with initial pacing set at 10–15 bpm higher than the ventricular rate to ensure that the atria only are being paced. The electrocardiogram should be monitored during overdrive pacing and bipolar pacing used. The pacer is set to 20 mA (full current), and the rate is set at 10 bmp faster than the rate of flutter or tachycardia. After atrial capture, the rate is increased slowly until change occurs in flutter waves (usually at 20%–30% higher than the atrial flutter rate) with pacing continued for 1 minute; then the pacer is turned off immediately, and the patient's rate and rhythm are assessed. If the tachycardia converts to marked bradycardia, then the pacemaker may be set at about 60 mA until the sinus mechanism stabilizes.

Atrioventricular pacing

Atrioventricular (AV) pacing may shorten the AV delay typically found after cardiac surgery. To initiate AV pacing, both atrial and ventricular wires are attached to the AV pacer with both outlets set at 10–20 mA with a PR interval of 150 ms. With atrial activity, the DDD mode is used. Without atrial activity,

DDD or DVI modes can be used. AV pacing is indicated for heart block (i.e., complete, first-degree, second-degree). Patients who have normal conduction should have atrial pacing alone. AV pacing is usually better than ventricular pacing because the atria are important for filling and 20%–30% of cardiac output. Left ventricular systolic and diastolic functions are improved with biventricular pacing. Atrial fibrillation during AV pacing may be signaled by abrupt hemodynamic instability.

Ventricular pacing

Ventricular pacing increases the risk of atrial fibrillation (Afib), but it can be used to slow the ventricular response to Afib or when atrial pacing is unable to maintain an adequate heart rate or to overdrive ventricular tachycardia. To initiate ventricular pacing, both ventricular wires are connected to the pulse generator for bipolar pacing, or one wire is connected to the negative pole and a different electrode (e.g., an atrial wire) to the positive for unipolar pacing. The mode is set at VVI with a ventricular output of 10–20 mA in the demand (synchronous) mode. The sensing threshold must be monitored as undersensing may cause incorrect pacing, and oversensing may inhibit pacing. The rate is adjusted according to the problem for which pacing is initiated. Left ventricular systolic and diastolic functions are improved with biventricular pacing. Care must be taken that ventricular pacing wires are not inappropriately sensing as this can result in ventricular tachycardia (VT). VT is treated with rapid ventricular pacing.

Pacemaker syndrome

Pacemaker syndrome can occur with any type of pacemaker if there is inadequate synchronicity between the contractions of the atria and ventricles, resulting in a decrease in cardiac output, and inadequate atrial contribution to the filling of ventricles. Total peripheral vascular resistance may increase to maintain blood pressure, but hypotension occurs if it decreases.

Mild	Pulsations evident in neck and abdomen Cardiac palpitations Headache and feeling of anxiety General malaise and unexplained weakness Pain or "fullness" in the jaw or chest
Moderate	Increasing dyspnea on exertion with accompanying orthopnea Dizziness, vertigo, and increasing confusion Feeling of choking
Severe	Increasing pulmonary edema with dyspnea even at rest and crackling rales Syncope Heart failure

Pacemaker complications

Pacemakers, transvenous, temporary, and permanent, are invasive foreign bodies and as such can cause a number of different complications.

Infection, bleeding, or hematoma may occur at the entry site of leads for temporary pacemakers or at the subcutaneous area of implantation for permanent generators. Puncture of the subclavian vein or internal mammary artery may cause a hemothorax. The endocardial electrode may irritate the ventricular wall, causing ectopic beats or tachycardia.

Dislodgement of the transvenous lead may lead to malfunction or perforation of the myocardium. This is one of the most common early complications.

Dislocation of leads may result in phrenic nerve or muscle stimulation (which may be evidenced by hiccupping).

Cardiac tamponade may result when epicardial wires of temporary pacing are removed.

General malfunctioning of the pacemaker may indicate dislodgement, dislocation, interference caused by electromagnetic fields, and the need for new batteries or generator.

Pacemaker syndrome may result.

<u>Undersensing and oversensing</u>

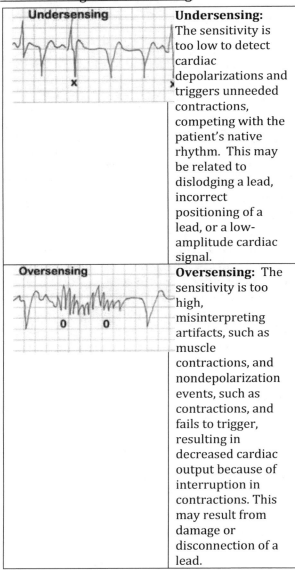

Undersensing	**Undersensing:** The sensitivity is too low to detect cardiac depolarizations and triggers unneeded contractions, competing with the patient's native rhythm. This may be related to dislodging a lead, incorrect positioning of a lead, or a low-amplitude cardiac signal.
Oversensing	**Oversensing:** The sensitivity is too high, misinterpreting artifacts, such as muscle contractions, and nondepolarization events, such as contractions, and fails to trigger, resulting in decreased cardiac output because of interruption in contractions. This may result from damage or disconnection of a lead.

Noncapture

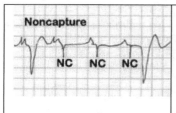 Noncapture NC NC NC	**Noncapture:** The pacemaker does not trigger contractions. This may be related to settings, lead disconnection, low battery, or metabolic changes.

Troubleshooting methods for problems associated with epicardial pacing

Non-functioning	Wires may be defective or connections faulty. Electrodes may not be positioned properly or may have become dislodged. Atrial fibrillation may be occurring and causing atrial capture to fail. Battery may be low.
Threshold changes	Changes in condition (e.g., edema, inflammation, scar tissue near electrodes, thrombus formation) may cause the threshold to rise after surgery. If heart block continues for a number of days, a permanent transvenous pacemaker may need to be inserted.
Oversensing	In DDD pacing, atrial fibrillation and flutter may result in a fast ventricular rate. The upper rate should be programmed lower or the pacemaker mode changed to VVI. VVI pacing may be inhibited by oversensing T waves.
Ventricular tachycardia (VT)/ ventricular fibrillation(VF)	Asynchronous ventricular pacing may trigger VT/VF. Ventricular pacing must be done in demand mode, and unused wires should be isolated and capped so they do not inadvertently trigger contractions.
Mediastinal bleeding	Mechanical irritation of the bypass graft can occur if wires are placed too close to surgical areas. Additionally, bleeding can occur from the atrial and ventricular surfaces where the wires are secured if the sutures are too tight or near small vessels. Pacing wires should not be removed until heparin is discontinued and INR is stable to reduce the chance of bleeding. Patients must be monitored carefully for cardiac tamponade.
Competing rhythm	Atrial or ventricular ectopic beats may occur with asynchronous pacing if the pacemaker's rate is too close to the patient's intrinsic rate. Turning the pacemaker off should relieve this situation.
Difficulty in removing wires	If pacing wires are secured too tightly or get caught under other sutures or wires, they may dislodge easily. Holding loose traction may help to dislodge the wires, but if this is not successful, the wire should be pulled out gently as far as possible and cut off at the skin. Once cut and the traction stopped, the wire should retract.

Intraaortic Balloon Pump

Use

The intra-aortic balloon pump (IABP) is the most commonly used circulatory assist device. The IABP improves hemodynamic status and controls and prevents ischemia pre- and postoperatively.

Indications

Indications include the following:
- Postsurgical left ventricular failure and low cardiac output
- Unstable angina
- Refractory ischemia and hemodynamic instability
- Myocardial infarction with complications or persistent angina
- Cardiogenic shock
- Papillary muscle dysfunction or rupture with mitral regurgitation or ventricular septal rupture
- Nonresponsive ventricular dysrhythmias
- Contraindications include aortic regurgitation or dissection and severe atherosclerosis (aortic/peripheral)

Insertion

The intra-aortic balloon pump (IABP) is a catheter with an inflatable balloon from the tip and lengthwise down the catheter. The catheter is usually inserted through the femoral artery but may be placed during surgery or through a cut-down. The catheter is threaded into the descending thoracic aorta, and the balloon inflates distal to the left subclavian artery during diastole to increase circulation to the coronary arteries; it then deflates during systole to decrease afterload.

Removal

Anticoagulation is reduced and usually discontinued before removal of the IABP. When an IABP is removed percutaneously, initial pressure is applied distal to the insertion site for a few heartbeats to flush out the wound. Pressure is then applied slightly proximal to the insertion site as the artery puncture site is slightly cephalad to the skin puncture site. Steady pressure should be maintained for 45 minutes or more without interruption to prevent the formation of thrombus. The D-STAT dry hemostatic bandage, which contains bovine thrombin, may be used to improve surface hemostasis.

Complications

Complications associated with an intra-aortic balloon pump (IABP) include the following:
- Dysrhythmias (may interfere with ballooning)
- Peripheral ischemia from femoral artery occlusion
- Balloon perforation or rupture, requiring immediate removal; migration; or inadequate ballooning
- Vascular injury, including aortic dissection/rupture, thrombosis, vascular occlusion, and embolization
- Renal ischemia if the balloon is placed too distally
- Thrombocytopenia from damage to circulating platelets, so a daily platelet count is necessary
- Distal ischemia is the most common complication, so distal pulses/Doppler signals must be assessed routinely. Ischemia may result from thrombosis near the site of insertion. Ischemia is most common in those with prolonged IABP use and in older female patients, diabetics, and patients with preexisting peripheral vascular disease. Cool extremities in the initial postoperative period may result from hypothermia, peripheral vasoconstriction, or low cardiac output, but this should reverse with treatment

Balloon inflation and deflation timing

The timing of balloon inflation and deflation with the intra-aortic balloon pump (IABP) is done using the electrocardiogram (ECG) or arterial waveform:

- ECG: Inflation occurs at the peak of the T wave, and deflation occurs before or on the R wave
- Arterial waveform: Inflation occurs at the dichrotic notch, and deflation occurs just before the aortic upstroke

Most commonly the ECG is used as a trigger; the R wave indicates ventricular systole, and the arterial waveform is used to determine timing. Initially, the setting of inflation is 1:2 with every other heartbeat receiving assistance for comparison purposes. Then, the timing is set at 1:1 or other settings as needed by the patient. Criteria for optimal inflation include the following:

- Distinct V-shape occurs at the dicrotic notch
- Augmented diastolic pressure is more than or equal to the previous systolic pressure.

Criteria for optimal deflation include:

- Assisted end-diastolic pressure is 5–10 mm Hg lower than the unassisted end-diastolic pressure
- Assisted systolic pressure is 5–10 mm Hg lower than unassisted systolic pressure

Timing errors

While timing is carried out automatically, waveforms should be monitored carefully as manual adjustments may be required. Equipment varies, so manufacturer's directions should always be consulted. Correctly timing inflation is especially important. Timing errors with the intra-aortic balloon pump include early or late inflation and deflation.

Early inflation
Early inflation is aortic regurgitation from early valve closing and decreased stroke volume, increasing end-diastolic volume and the need for myocardial oxygen (waveform loses V shape).

Late inflation
Late inflation id decreased coronary artery perfusion pressures (diastolic augmentation after dicrotic notch).

Early deflation
Early deflation is increased afterload and need for myocardial oxygen (sharp drop-off in waveform with U curve before systolic upstroke).

Late deflation
Late deflation it the loss of afterload reduction as balloon blocks left ventricular ejection of blood (systolic waveform widened and slow rise in the next assisted systole).

Weaning criteria

When the intra-aortic balloon pump (IABP) is initially placed, the inflation ratio is usually set at 1:2, with alternate beats assisted, but this may be changed to 1:1 if necessary. The ratio may be decreased to 1:3 or 1:4 or more as the patient's condition improves and is weaned from the IABP. Weaning criteria include the following:

- Normal or acceptable serum lactate, electrolytes, and hemoglobin/hematocrit levels
- Absence of chest pain, dyspnea, or indications of decreased cerebral perfusion (e.g., confusion, restlessness, anxiety, altered mental status)
- Normal or near-normal heart rate without significant dysrhythmia

Stable hemodynamic status:

- Mean arterial pressure over 65–70 mm Hg
- Pulmonary artery occlusion pressure less than 18 mm Hg

- Cardiac index over 2 L/min/m^2
- Systemic vascular resistance less than 2000 dynes/sec/cm^{-5}
- Urinary output over 0.5 mL/kg/hr
- Venous oxygen saturation 60%–80%

Both the ratio of assisted beats and the amount of gas in the balloon are decreased during weaning. Gas volume is usually reduced about 20% at each step in the weaning process; however, volume reduction increases the risk of thrombus formation, so the ratio is decreased more rapidly.

Monitoring patients

Monitoring patients with intra-aortic balloon pumps (IABPs) involves checking the hemodynamic status every 15 minutes initially, then hourly, and then as indicated. The electrocardiogram and chest x-ray are performed daily, and intravenous therapy is maintained to ensure adequate preload. IABP settings must be checked and documented hourly with a waveform tracing printed every 12 hours or with changes. Distal pulses and sensorimotor function are checked every 15–30 minutes and then every hour; an ankle-brachial index is checked every 4 hours. A left radial pulse is monitored as an absence indicates upward migration of the catheter. Heparin levels are maintained with anticoagulation studies every 6 hours. Respiratory status is monitored every 4 hours with incentive spirometry every 2 hours, and the head of bed is maintained at 30°–45° to prevent aspiration. Patients should be advised to avoid flexing the hip on the affected side and may need a leg immobilizer. Patients should be log rolled for skin care.

ABI procedure

The ankle-brachial index (ABI) examination is done to evaluate peripheral arterial disease of the lower extremities.

Apply blood pressure cuff to one arm, palpate brachial pulse, and place conductivity gel over the artery.

Place the tip of a Doppler device at a 45° angle into the gel at the brachial artery, and listen for the pulse sound.

Inflate the cuff until the pulse sound ceases, and then inflate the cuff 20 mm Hg above that point.

Release air, and listen for the return of the pulse sound. This reading is the brachial systolic pressure.

Repeat the procedure on the other arm, and use the higher reading for calculations.

Repeat the same procedure on each ankle with the cuff applied above the malleoli and the gel over the posterior tibial pulse to obtain the ankle systolic pressure.

Divide the ankle systolic pressure by the brachial systolic pressure to obtain the ABI. Sometimes, readings are taken both before and after 5 minutes of walking on a treadmill.

Interpreting the results
Once the ankle-brachial index (ABI) examination is completed, the ankle systolic pressure must be divided by the brachial systolic pressure. Ideally, the blood pressure at the ankle should be equal to that of the arm or slightly higher. With peripheral arterial disease, the ankle pressure falls, affecting the ABI. Additionally, some conditions that cause calcification of arteries, such as diabetes, can cause a false elevation. Calculation is simple: If the ankle systolic pressure is 90 mm Hg and the brachial systolic pressure is 120 mm Hg, then 90/120 = .75. The degree of disease relates to the score.

Ankle-brachial Index Score	
> 1.3	Abnormally high, may indicate calcification of vessel wall
1–1.1	Normal reading, asymptomatic
< 0.95	Indicates narrowing of one or more leg blood vessels
< 0.8	Moderate, often associated with intermittent claudication during exercise
< 0.6–0.8	Borderline perfusion
0.5–0.75	Severe disease, ischemia
< 0.5	Pain even at rest and limb threatened
0.25	Critical limb-threatening condition

Short-term mechanical circulation devices

Short-term mechanical circulation devices may be used for an emergent bridge to transplant. These include the Abiomed pumps, which require sternotomy and can be used for right, left, or bilateral ventricular support. The TandemHeart PTVA system is inserted percutaneously into the femoral vein and threaded to the left atrium. Oxygenated blood from the left atrium is returned to the femoral artery by an arterial cannula. This device has been used to treat cardiogenic shock after cardiotomy. Extracorporeal membrane oxygenation may also be used for days or weeks, oxygenating the blood while bypassing the heart and lungs.

VADS

Ventricular assist devises (VADs) can provide support to the left ventricle (most common), right ventricle, or both. With most devices, blood drains from the base of the left ventricle into the pump through an inflow cannula and back into the aorta through an outflow cannula. The pump is placed preperitoneally in the abdomen with electrical cables and an air vent tunneled through a percutaneous line to the external controller. Left VADs require good right ventricular function.

Indications

In some cases after cardiac surgery, patients cannot be weaned from cardiopulmonary bypass even with medications and use of an intra-aortic bypass pump. In that case, a ventricular assist device (VAD) may be inserted. Other indications include acute myocardial infarction with cardiogenic shock, metabolic abnormalities, and a cardiac index less than 1.8 L/min/m².

Left VAD (LVAD) decompresses the left ventricle and provides systemic perfusion. Systolic blood pressure is less than 90 mm Hg, left atrial pressure is more than 20 mm Hg, and systemic vascular resistance is more than 2100 dynes/cm⁵, with decreased urinary output of less than 20 mL/hr.

Right VAD (RVAD) decompresses the right ventricle and provides pulmonary blood flow. Mean right atrial pressure is more than 20 mm Hg, left atrial pressure is less than 15 mm Hg, and there is no indication of tricuspid regurgitation.

Right and left VAD (BiVAD) provides both systemic and pulmonary blood flow support. Left atrial pressure is more than 20 mm Hg, right atrial pressure is more than 20–25 mm Hg, and there is no tricuspid regurgitation. For those with LVAD, the BiVAD is indicated if the LVAD cannot maintain flow more than 2 L min/m² with right atrial pressure more than 20 mm Hg.

Monitoring of the patient

After the insertion of a ventricular assist device (VAD), the patient must be monitored carefully.

To avoid infection, dressings over drive-line exit sites must be changed daily and the drainage and wound conditions noted. Any changes in temperature (< 36°C or > 28.5°C) or erythema, purulent discharge, foul odor, or skin separation must be reported immediately.

Trauma is prevented by applying abdominal binders to secure the cannulas.

Albumin levels must be monitored (maintain > 2.5 g/dL) to promote healing.

Right ventricular (RV) failure, including right arterial pressure and central venous pressure, may occur in which case RV support (dobutamine, 3–5 mcg/kg/min, or milrinone, 0.135–0.375 mcg/kg/min) must be provided. Nitric oxide may also improve RV function.

Renal function for patients with left VAD must be monitored as renal function may decrease postoperatively, especially with heart failure.

Hepatic function must be monitored for patients with heart failure or those who received intraoperative transfusions.

Mediastinal Drainage

Mediastinal bleeding

Mediastinal bleeding that is directly associated with the surgery with a normal coagulation profile is classified as surgical bleeding, while bleeding associated with coagulopathies is classified as medical bleeding. When bleeding occurs, identifying and treating the underlying cause is critical. Causes can include a residual or rebound heparin effect, excessive protamine, thrombocytopenia or platelet dysfunction, deficiency in clotting factor, and fibrinolysis.

Risk factors
A number of risk factors may increase the risk of postsurgical mediastinal bleeding:

- Older age and patients with small body surface area (especially females)
- History of anemia and advanced cardiac disease, especially with left ventricular dysfunction

- History of kidney or liver disease, diabetes, peripheral vascular disease, and coagulopathies
- Medications (preoperative), including high-dose aspirin, low-molecular-weight heparin (≤ 18 hours), fondaparinux (≤ 48 hours), clopidogrel, prasugrel, IIb/IIIA inhibitors, thrombolytic treatment before emergent surgery, and an incomplete INR reversal for patients on warfarin
- Complex, emergent, or repeat operations and use of an internal thoracic artery graft

Postoperative mediastinal bleeding

Excessive postoperative mediastinal bleeding occurs in 3%–14% of cardiac patients. Changing the patient's position may cause increased chest tube drainage because of pooling of blood. Acute onset of bleeding is characterized by bright red blood and continuous steady discharge. Dark red blood suggests older blood rather than active bleeding, especially if discharge slows after an initial increase. Bleeding may be surgical (bleeding from vessel or sutures) or nonsurgical (related to coagulopathy). Chest tube drainage should not exceed 200 mL in 2–6 hours. Excessive bleeding may require coagulation studies, a repeat chest x-ray to evaluate the width of the mediastinum, and transesophageal echocardiogram if cardiac tamponade is suspected. Indications for emergent surgical exploration include the following situations:

- Blood loss of more than 400 mL/hr for 4 hours
- Blood loss of 300 mL/hr for 3 hours
- Blood loss of 400 mL/hr for 2 hours
- Blood loss of 500 mL/hr for 1 hour

Treatment for coagulopathy may include fresh frozen plasma, platelets, cryoprecipitate, packed red blood cells, desmopressin to improve platelet function, aminocaproic acid to prevent fibrinolysis, and factor VIIa to help achieve hemostasis.

Treatment options

Treatment for mediastinal bleeding associated with coagulopathies varies, depending on the underlying problem. Routine point-of-care testing of coagulation is indicated after cardiac surgery to help determine the cause of bleeding:

- Increased activated clotting time more than 130 seconds and increased partial thromboplastin time more than 1.5 x normal: protamine, 2550 mg, initially although reinfusing cell-saver blood may reintroduce heparin and result in heparin-rebound effect, so may need continuous infusion at low dose or repeat doses
- Thrombocytopenia less than 100,000/mm^3 or platelet dysfunction (common in patients who are markedly anemic or have undergone cardiopulmonary bypass): administration of platelet transfusions; without bleeding, platelet transfusions not indicated until the level falls to 20,000–30,000/mm^3 (although most patients bleed at 50,000–60,000/mm^3)
- INR over 1.5: administration of fresh frozen plasma
- Fibrinogen less than 100 mg/dL: administration of cryoprecipitate
- Increased prothrombin time: fresh frozen plasma, cryoprecipitate, or both

Emergent Reopening of the Chest

Indications

An hourly bleeding rate of more than 400 mL in 1 hour indicates the need for emergent reopening of the chest. Reopening should be considered any time there is a sudden onset of excessive bleeding (> 300 mL/hr) because delay is associated with increased morbidity and death, increased need for transfusions, hemodynamic instability, and the risk of cardiac arrest. Other indications for emergent reopening of the chest include signs of cardiac tamponade and bleeding criteria:

- More than 300 mL/hr for 2–3 hours
- More than 200 mL/hr for 4 hours

Emergent resternotomy is also indicated for those who cannot be resuscitated after cardiac arrest, within 10 minutes of arrest, and tamponade with impending cardiac arrest. Because emergent sternotomy may be necessary after minimally invasive procedures, sternal saws should be available for emergencies. Resternotomy can be done up to 10 days after surgery.

Resternotomy procedure

A sternotomy surgical pack should be available at all times for cardiac surgery patients in addition to all necessary surgical equipment (e.g., drapes, antiseptics, cauterizers) and personal protective equipment (e.g., gowns, gloves, face masks). The resternotomy procedure includes the following:

- Apply ground pads for electrocautery device to patient's skin
- Remove sternal dressing, and pour antiseptic on patient's skin
- Apply draping
- Open wound with scalpel, and cut sternal wires with wire cutters
- Expose the heart with sternal retractors
- Suction and control bleeding as indicated
- Carry out manual massage or internal defibrillation as indicated
- Irrigate the mediastinum with warm normal saline or antibiotic solution
- Close the sternum
- Secure epicardial pacing wires, and apply protective dressing
- Secure chest tubes
- Upon closure of the wound, the patient must be monitored for hemodynamic status at least every 15 minutes until

the patient's condition stabilizes. Assessment of the chest tube drainage, wound, coagulation, and hematology should be ongoing

Assist with Internal Defibrillation

Internal defibrillation

Internal defibrillation for life-threatening ventricular tachycardia/ventricular fibrillation that does not respond to external defibrillation requires that the chest is opened similar to emergent resternotomy and that advanced cardiac life support is initiated. Sterile internal defibrillator paddles are prepared, and the paddles are placed on the heart, one over the right side (atrium or ventricle) and the other over the heart apex. The paddles are charged to 5–20 joules (usually 20 joules), and all employees are reminded to stand clear of the patient and equipment during defibrillation. Upon completion, the patient is assessed for conversion to sinus rhythm or the presence of a pulse. If no conversion occurs or the patient remains pulseless, then defibrillation is repeated. If the pericardium has not been opened, the repeat defibrillations may be done at 40 and 60 joules, but 20 joules is the recommended maximum if the pericardium is removed.

Cardiac arrest

Cardiac arrest may occur during cardiac surgery or in the postoperative period. Management includes the following:

- Establish airway, and manually ventilate with positive pressure ventilation at a rate of 8–10 breaths/min
- Provide chest compressions at 100/min after three attempts at defibrillation for ventricular tachycardia (VT)/ventricular

fibrillation (VF) or pacing for asystole. Perform until stable or the chest can be opened
- For VT/VF that is not responsive to defibrillation, perform cardiopulmonary resuscitation (CPR), and give epinephrine, 1 mg, and vasopressin, 40 U
- For recurrent VT/VF after three shocks, give amiodarone, 300 mg; lidocaine, 1–1.5 mg/kg bolus; or both, and give magnesium sulfate, 1–2 g in 10 mL 5% dextrose in water for torsades de pointes/hypermagnesemia. Give a single shock every 2 minutes until resternotomy

Cardiac arrest may occur during cardiac surgery or in the postoperative period. Management includes the following:

- When asystole is not responsive to pacing, give atropine, 3 mg, and perform external pacing and CPR until resternotomy
- Perform defibrillation for ventricular fibrillation and pulseless ventricular tachycardia. Emergency sternotomy should be done within 10 minutes of arrest if other methods are ineffective
- Assess for cause (e.g., cardiac tamponade, hypovolemia, pacing failure, pneumothorax, myocardial infarction). Provide oxygen with facemask, and intubate. Review chest tube drainage, x-rays, medications, and doses, and evaluate the cardiac monitor and the electrocardiogram

Causes
Cardiac arrest may result from a number of different causes:

- Acidosis (hydrogen ion): Administer sodium bicarbonate
- Hypovolemia: Fluid resuscitation is necessary to maintain fluid balance and increase blood pressure
- Hypoxia: Patients should receive hand ventilation with supplementary oxygen at 100%

- Potassium imbalance: Administer calcium chloride, glucose, insulin, bicarbonate for hyperkalemia, and an infusion of potassium chloride for hypokalemia
- Hypothermia: Use warming blankets, and increase ambient temperature as indicated
- Cardiac tamponade: Perform pericardiocentesis or emergent sternotomy
- Pneumothorax (tension): Perform a needle decompression and insertion of chest tube
- Myocardial infarction: Perform emergent cardiac catheterization, intra-aortic balloon pump, and treatment as indicated
- Pulmonary embolism: Administer oxygen and anticoagulant. Embolectomy or an inferior vena cava umbrella may be indicated
- Medications: Overdose of drugs may require activated charcoal and gastric lavage or antidote. Treat digoxin toxicity with digoxin immune Fab (Digibind). Treat toxicity from β-blockers and calcium channel blockers with inotropes and pacing

Ventilator Management

Negative inspiratory pressure

Negative inspiratory pressure is the pressure generated in a forced inspiration with obstructed airflow. It assesses the patient's ability to cough hard enough to mobilize and expel secretions.

Tidal volume

Tidal volume is the volume of air expelled with normal exhalation (not forced).

Minute ventilation

Minute ventilation is the volume of gas exchange (including both inhaled and exhaled) in 1 minute.

IPS

Intrapulmonary shunt (IPS) is the percentage of cardiac output that does not go through gas exchange because it does not come in contact with ventilated alveoli. This may result from atelectasis or hypoxemia after cardiac surgery. The usual intrapulmonary shunt is 5% or less, although those with acute respiratory distress syndrome may have shunts up to 50%. Oxygen is not effective in treating IPS.

Alveolar-arterial (A-a) oxygen gradient

Alveolar-arterial (A-a) oxygen gradient is the difference in the percentage of alveolar oxygen and the percentage of arterial oxygen. The A-a gradient can help to identify the cause of hypoxemia and to identify IPS. A simplified formula is:
- $PAO_2 - PaO_2$

Primary respiratory function

The body's cells obtain energy from the oxidation of carbohydrates, fats, and proteins, a process that requires oxygen and generates carbon dioxide as a by-product. The primary respiratory function is to facilitate this process:

Oxygen transport	Blood circulates to carry oxygen to the cells and to remove carbon dioxide by diffusion at the capillary level.
Respiration	Gas exchange occurs between the atmospheric air and the blood and between the blood and the body cell. The capillaries in the lungs have a lower concentration of oxygen than the alveoli, so oxygen diffuses into the blood. The capillaries have a higher concentration of carbon dioxide than the alveoli, so carbon dioxide diffuses into the alveoli.
Ventilation	Air flows into the lungs during inspiration and back into the atmosphere during expiration with airflow governed by variances in air pressure, airway resistance, and compliance.

Factors related to ventilation

Air pressure variances	Inspiration: The thorax expands and lowers the pressure in the thoracic cavity relative to atmospheric pressure, drawing air into the alveoli. Expiration: The diaphragm relaxes, the lungs contract, and pressure inside the alveoli increases relative to atmospheric pressure, causing air to flow out of the lungs.
Airway resistance	Resistance directly relates to the size of the airway, so changes in size can increase resistance, requiring an increased effort of breathing: Bronchial contraction, smooth muscles (asthma) Mucosal hyperplasia (chronic bronchitis) Airway obstruction (tumor, mucus, foreign body) Dilation, loss of elasticity (chronic obstructive pulmonary disease [COPD])
Compliance	The elasticity and expandability of the lungs and thoracic cavity determine the volume/pressure relationship: Compliance decreases when lung expansion is limited or "tight" (e.g., pneumothorax, pulmonary edema, atelectasis, acute respiratory distress disorder), requiring an increased effort of breathing. Compliance increases with

Oxygen administration related terms

Flow rate (FR)	The FR is the number of liters of oxygen flow per minute. During titration, flow may be adjusted, according to the patient's response by using the least amount required to obtain optimal oxygen saturation.
Fraction of inspired oxygen (FiO₂)	The FiO₂ is the percentage of oxygen in the mixture of air provided to the patient. This ranges from that of room air, 21%, to 100%, but is usually maintained at less than 60%. FiO₂ may be expressed as a decimal or percentage: 0.50 equals 50%. When ordering oxygen for titration, the physician may not specify the exact FiO₂ but rather the target oxygen saturation.
Liters per minute (LPM)	LPM measures the liters of oxygen administered.
Room air (RA)	RA is 21% oxygen. This is the usual air provided by positive airway pressure.

Oxyhemoglobin dissociation curve

The oxyhemoglobin dissociation curve is a graph that plots the percentage of hemoglobin saturated with oxygen (Y axis) and different partial pressures of oxygen

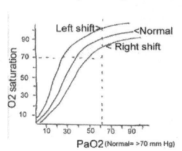

(PaO₂ levels) [X axis]. A curve shift to the right, as occurs with acidosis, represents conditions where hemoglobin has less affinity for oxygen, and greater amounts of oxygen are released into the tissues. Low pH shifts the curve to the right, enabling increased off-loading of hemoglobin to tissues. A shift to the left, which occurs with hypothermia and alkalosis, has the opposite implications, increased binding of oxygen but less release to the tissues. Blood transfusions and elevated oxygen shifts the

curve to the left, causing increased affinity of hemoglobin for oxygen in the lungs. Normal PaO₂ is 80–100 mm Hg, equal to 95%–98% oxygen saturation. Levels less than 40 mm Hg are dangerous.

Arterial oxygen

Arterial oxygen is carried in the red blood cells by hemoglobin. Each hemoglobin molecule can carry four molecules of oxygen, with 1 g of hemoglobin equal to 1.39 mL of oxygen (100 mL arterial blood carries 0.3 mL oxygen). When the hemoglobin is fully saturated (4 oxygen molecules per molecule of hemoglobin), then arterial oxygen saturation is 100%. A small amount of oxygen remains dissolved in blood (partial pressure of oxygen [PaO₂] x 0.003), but this has little effect on arterial oxygen content. The formula to determine arterial oxygen (CaO₂) is described below:
- CaO₂ = (hemoglobin x arterial oxygen saturation [SaO₂] x 1.39) + (PaO₂ x 0.003)

A simplified formula is sometimes used to evaluate oxygen delivery (O₂D):
- O₂D = (stroke volume x heart rate) x oxygen saturation (SpO₂)

Perfusion pressure is estimated by the systolic blood pressure:
- Systolic blood pressure = cardiac output x systemic vascular resistance

Because the oxygen in the blood is related to hemoglobin levels, correcting anemia more effectively increases PaO₂ than increasing the fraction of inspired oxygen.

PaCO₂ Factors

There are many factors that can affect the partial pressure of carbon dioxide (PaCO₂) level in the blood, including conditions that relate to respiratory acidosis and metabolic alkalosis:

- Increased $PaCO_2$ and acute respiratory acidosis may occur with central nervous system depression caused by medications (e.g., sedatives), stroke, head trauma, neuromuscular diseases (e.g., Guillain-Barré, myasthenia gravis, muscular dystrophy), lung disorders (e.g., pleural effusion, pneumothorax), airway obstruction, and acute respiratory disorders (e.g., pneumonia, hyperventilation, pulmonary edema)
- Increased $PaCO_2$ and chronic respiratory acidosis may occur with chronic disorders, such as chronic obstructive pulmonary disease, kyphoscoliosis, and scleroderma
- Decreased $PaCO_2$ and metabolic alkalosis may occur with diabetic ketoacidosis, uremia, hyperalbuminemia, ethyl alcohol ingestion, salicylate poisoning, hypokalemia, uretero-sigmoidostomy, renal tubular acidosis, angiotensin-converting enzyme inhibitors, and hyperkalemia
- Increased $PaCO_2$ to 70 mm Hg is an indication of imminent respiratory failure, requiring intubation. This is especially true if the $PaCO_2$ is rebounding from a previous lack of carbon dioxide in the arterial sampling. This is common in hyperventilating asthmatics who are tiring and headed for respiratory arrest

Prolonged postoperative ventilation need indicators

Preoperative	**Preexisting conditions:** diabetes, recent myocardial infarction, pulmonary edema, previous cardiac surgery, peripheral vascular disease, left ventricular impairment with an ejection fraction of less than 40%, increased serum creatinine, cardiogenic shock, sepsis, chronic obstructive pulmonary disease, class III or IV congestive heart failure, aortic aneurysm, valvular disease, and need for intubation. **Age and gender:** 75 years of age or older and female
Intraoperative	Deep hypothermic circulatory arrest, prolonged cardiopulmonary bypass over 4–6 hours, extended duration of surgery, abnormal serum glucose levels, coagulopathy, multiple procedures, perioperative heart failure, and severe myocardial dysfunction
Postoperative	Impaired mentation, excessive mediastinal bleeding, hemodynamic instability, need for intra-aortic balloon pump, pulmonary edema, hypoxia, respiratory failure, stroke, parenteral nutrition, acute respiratory distress syndrome, and need for inotropic agents or transfusions

Postoperative ventilator settings

Postoperative ventilator settings include:
- Type of ventilation: synchronized intermittent mandatory ventilation, assist control, pressure support, or pressure control
- Control mode: controlled ventilation, assisted ventilation, synchronized intermittent mandatory (allows spontaneous breaths between ventilator controlled inhalation/exhalation), positive end-expiratory pressure (PEEP) [positive pressure at end of expiration],

continuous positive airway pressure, and bilevel positive airway pressure

- Tidal volume (Vt): set in relation to respiratory rate, 8–12 mL/kg ideal body weight. An increase may decrease carbon dioxide, and a decrease may increase carbon dioxide levels
- Inspiratory–expiratory ratio (I:E): ranges from 1:2 but may vary
- Respiratory rate: depends on Vt and partial pressure of carbon dioxide ($PaCO_2$) target, 8–18 breaths/min
- Fraction of inspired oxygen (FiO_2): the percentage of oxygen in the inspired air, usually ranges from 21%–100% and maintained at less than 40% to avoid toxicity; depends on arterial blood gas and oxygen saturation (0.4–1.0)
- Sensitivity: determines the effort needed to trigger inspiration
- Pressure: controls the pressure exerted in delivering Vt, 5–10 cm H_2O
- Rate of inspiratory flow: controls the liters per minute speed of Vt, 30–60 L/min
- Minute volume: 100–120
- PEEP: 5–10 cm H_2O

Mechanical ventilation

Complicaton prevention
Methods to prevent complications from mechanical ventilation include:

- Elevate the patient's head and chest to 30° to prevent aspiration and ventilation-associated pneumonia
- Reposition patient every 2 hours
- Provide deep venous thrombosis prophylaxis, such as external compression support or heparin (5000 U subcutaneously two to three times daily)
- Administer famotidine (20 mg twice a day by nasogastric [NG] tube or intravenously [IV]) or sucralfate (1 g per NG tube four times day) to prevent gastrointestinal bleeding

- Decrease and eliminate sedation/analgesia as soon as possible
- Follow careful protocols for pressure settings to prevent barotrauma. Tidal volumes are usually maintained at 8–10 mL/kg ideal body weight
- Monitor for pneumothorax or evidence of barotrauma
- Conduct nutritional assessment (including lab tests) to prevent malnutrition
- Monitor intake and output carefully, and administer IV fluids to prevent dehydration
- Do daily spontaneous breathing trials, and discontinue ventilation as soon as possible

Modes

Control mode (CM)	Inspiration and expiration as well as tidal volume (Vt) and rate are preset, and the patient cannot initiate breaths or alter pattern. This mode is rarely used, and patients may require sedation to prevent competition with ventilation.
Continuous mandatory ventilation (CMV)	The Vt and rate are preset, but the patient can initiate breaths but cannot alter the Vt. This is frequently used after anesthesia. Patients may need sedation to decrease spontaneous breaths.
Synchronized intermittent mandatory ventilation (SIMV)	The Vt and rate are preset and synchronized with the patient's spontaneous breathing in this primary ventilation mode. This mode is often used to wean patients from the ventilator. Respiration rates of less than 6 breaths/min can cause increased work of breathing.
Pressure support ventilation (PSV)	Positive pressure is supplied during spontaneous inspiration. This mode does not have a preset rate, so patients must be monitored closely for fatigue or apnea. This mode is used for higher pressures and to wean patients with chronic obstructive pulmonary disease.

Clinical judgment (pulmonary)

Ventilator weaning
Ventilator weaning has three phases: removal of the ventilator, extubation, and finally removal of supportive oxygen. Criteria for ventilator weaning in the early postoperative period include the following:

- Patient awake without stimulation, not shivering, and able to grip hand or lift head for 5 seconds
- Neuromuscular blockade reversal evident and patient moving
- Core temperature stable at 35.5°C or higher
- Stable systolic blood pressure of 100–140 mm Hg
- Heart rate stable at less than 120 bpm without arrhythmias
- Cardiac index 2.2 L/min/m^2 or more
- Chest tube drainage less than 50–100 mL/hr
- Minute ventilation of about 6 L/min (respiratory rate x tidal volume)
- Rapid shallow breath index less than 100 breaths/min/L
- Partial pressure of oxygen (PaO_2)/fraction of inspired oxygen (FiO_2) more than 150 ($PaO_2 > 75$ torr on FiO_2 of 0.5)
- Partial pressure of carbon dioxide ($PaCO_2$) less than 50 torr
- pH 7.3–7.5

Ventilator weaning criteria
When patients have been on prolonged ventilation, the underlying disease process should be stable, and the patient should be awake and alert enough to breathe independently. Hemodynamic status should be stable with no vasoactive drugs, and hemoglobin and metabolic status satisfactory. Arterial blood gases should be stable with a respiratory rate less than 35 breaths/min and rapid shallow breathing index of less than 100. Criteria for oxygen weaning: FiO_2 is reduced until PaO_2 is 70–100 mm Hg on room air. Supplemental oxygen is necessary with a PaO_2 of less than 70 mm Hg.

Extubation readiness

During extubation, the oxygen saturation should be 92%–94% or more on a fraction of inspired oxygen of 40% and a positive end-expiratory pressure of 5 cm H_2O.Methods used to determine readiness for extubation include:

- Compliance, resistance, oxygenation, pressure (CROP) index: This identifies parameters that predict extubation success based on respiratory rate, compliance, arterial oxygen, maximum inspiratory pressure, and relative inspiratory effort
- Intermittent mandatory ventilation (IMV)/synchronized IMV (SIMV): The rate of ventilation is gradually reduced
- Pressure support ventilation (PSV): Inspiratory support is gradually reduced. In some cases, a minimum tidal volume is set per ventilator-assisted breath. PSV may be combined with IMV/SIMV
- Spontaneous breathing trial (SBT): SBT is usually in the morning for a prescribed period (30–120 minutes) after the patient exhibits some spontaneous triggering of respirations, and sedation is reduced. The ventilator rate is adjusted to 0, and pressure support is decreased. The SBT is discontinued if respiratory distress occurs

Ventilation extubation criteria

Extubation from ventilation in the initial postoperative period should be done after the patient meets the weaning criteria. Extubation can be done from continuous positive air pressure (CPAP) or T-piece. Ventilation extubation criteria include the following:
Patient meets weaning criteria.
Patient is able to maintain an awake state without stimulation.
Respiratory mechanics are acceptable:

- Tidal volume is 5 mL/kg ideal body weight or more
- Negative inspiratory force is 25 cm H_2O or more
- Vital capacity is 10–15 mL/kg or more
- Respirations (spontaneous) are 24 breath/min or less
- Blood gases are acceptable (on ≤ 5 CPAP/pressure support ventilation)
- Partial pressure of oxygen is 70 torr or more (with a fraction of inspired oxygen of ≤ 0.5)
- Partial pressure of carbon dioxide is 48 torr or less
- pH is 7.32–7.45

After an extended period of ventilation, patients should meet the criteria related to respiratory mechanics and blood gases and should have a respiratory rate of 35 breaths/min or more without agitation or diaphoresis and should be mentally alert and able to cough. A **cuff leak of 110** or more should be present with the cuff deflated.

Ventilator extubation failure criteria

About 5% of cardiac surgical patients fail extubation. Failure criteria for ventilator extubation include the following:
- Decreased oxygen saturation of less than 90%
- Agitation, diaphoresis, or increased somnolence
- Change in systolic blood pressure by more than 20 mm Hg/min or a rise to 160 mm Hg or more
- Heart rate increase or decrease of more than 20% or tachycardia of 120 bpm
- Need for vasoactive medications to maintain status
- Development or worsening of arrhythmias. Increased respiratory rate of 10 breaths/min or a rise to 35 breaths/min or more for a 5-minute period
- Partial pressure of oxygen of less than 60 torr (with a fraction of inspired oxygen of 0.5)

- Partial pressure of carbon dioxide of more than 50 torr with a pH of less than 7.30 (indicating respiratory acidosis)

Patients who are agitated may require more sedation and prolonged ventilation with weaning attempted when patient is stabilized. Avoid extubation at night if intubation was difficult in the event reintubation is necessary. Older patients with a slow metabolism may awaken more slowly, but reversal agents (e.g., naloxone) should be avoided as use may markedly increase pain. Small amounts of a reversal agent may be indicated after 24–36 hours to determine if the patient has suffered a stroke or other impairment.

Airway clearance

Airway clearance, the ability to move secretions or foreign particles from the upper airway and prevent aspiration, depends on an intact and functioning mucociliary system and the ability to cough effectively. Mucus provides barrier protection to the tissues, and the cilia mechanically move mucus and particles upward. Inflammation, asthma, chronic obstructive pulmonary disease, cystic fibrosis (CF), and mechanical ventilation can alter the viscosity of the mucus and impair its effectiveness. CF, lung transplantation, mechanical irritation, and smoking can damage cilia. Patients with tracheotomies or mechanical ventilation tend to retain secretions, impairing the exchange of oxygen and increasing the effort required to breathe, leading to increased inflammation and infection that further impair lung function. Both increased and retained secretions lead to decreased forced expiratory volume (in 1 second) and higher mortality rates. Cough is impaired by mechanical ventilation as well as restrictive and obstructive respiratory diseases. Airway clearance measures include the following:
- Directed cough, chest physiotherapy (if not on ventilator)

- Positioning with head of bed elevated
- Suctioning as needed (limited to 5 seconds in duration)
- Antibiotics for infection
- Bronchodilators
- Airway clearance devices

Postextubation management

Patients must be monitored carefully postextubation. Management includes: Patients who did not exhibit a cuff leak during positive pressure ventilation with the cuff deflated may have laryngotracheal edema that can lead to obstruction of the upper airway, especially after several days of ventilation. Patients may need oxygen (humidified at 40%–70%) because of decreased compliance of the chest wall, atelectasis, and pain inhibiting deep breathing. Patients with inadequate oxygenation may require a nonrebreather mask with oxygen at 8–15 L/min.

Bilevel positive airway pressure, continuous positive airway pressure (CPAP), or intermittent positive pressure breathing should be used for several days after surgery as they expand the lungs better than incentive spirometry. CPAP with a nasal mask may be used for patients with cardiogenic pulmonary edema. Dysphagia may occur, especially in patients with ventilation for over 48 hours, putting them at risk for aspiration. When hemodynamically stable, intravenous furosemide is administered to promote diuresis. Adequate analgesia is critical for recovery. Antiembolism stockings or devices and early mobilization can prevent thromboembolism.

Antibiotics are needed for a positive sputum culture, and bronchodilators are needed for bronchospasm).

BiPAP

Bilevel positive airway pressure (BiPAP) devices deliver two levels of pressure, which can be preset. Inspiratory positive airway pressure (IPAP) is set at a higher level than expiratory positive airway pressure (EPAP). This allows for the pressure needed to open the airway during inspiration but reduces pressure to facilitate expiration. Typically, BiPAP devices do not compensate for altitude and can be used with humidification. Some have software and downloadable memory to generate reports of sleep events.

Spontaneously timed (BiPAP ST) devices have two pressure settings for each breath as well as settings for the number of respirations so that they can trigger inspiration if the respiratory rate falls below a preset level, an important consideration for central sleep apnea and other pulmonary disorders. Settings include spontaneous mode, which triggers increased pressure after the person attempts to breath, and timed mode, which triggers increased pressure to initiate respiration within a preset time. Autotritrating BiPAP devices are also available and can vary both IPAP and EPAP automatically as needed to promote adequate ventilation.

CPAP determination

All positive airway pressure devices have air blowers that deliver pressurized room air to an interface or mask. Pressure can be increased or decreased by adjusting the speed or the amount of airflow, with most machines generating pressure ranging from 2–20 cm water pressure. Carbon dioxide is expelled through a vent or nonrebreather valve on expiration. A wide range of equipment is available for continuous positive airway pressure (CPAP), starting with the most basic relatively inexpensive machines to expensive computerized equipment.

Basic CPAP machines may be large or small, but all have filters in the back and can be used with a variety of masks (e.g., oral, nasal, orofacial, nasal pillow). Some have built-in heated humidifiers, and all can be used with

- 129 -

cool passover or heated humidifiers. Many basic machines do not adjust for environmental factors, such as altitude, and many do not have an internal memory to generate sleep reports. Some may switch between 110 and 200 volts. Even basic machines allow for a gradual rise to selected pressure.

More sophisticated CPAP machines usually have software and downloadable memories and can provide reports regarding respiratory events. Altitude compensation is usually automatic.

Positive pressure ventilators

Positive pressure ventilators assist respiration by applying pressure directly to the airway, inflating the lungs, forcing expansion of the alveoli, and facilitating gas exchange. Generally, endotracheal intubation or tracheostomy is necessary to maintain positive pressure ventilation for extended periods.

Pressure cycled
This type of ventilation is usually used for short-term treatment after extubation. The intermittent positive pressure breathing machine is the most common type. This delivers a flow of air to a preset pressure and then cycles off. Airway resistance or changes in compliance can affect the volume of air and may compromise ventilation.

Time cycled
This type of ventilation regulates the volume of air the patient receives by controlling the length of inspiration and the flow rate.

Volume cycled
This type of ventilation provides a preset flow of pressurized air during inspiration and then cycles off and allows passive expiration, providing a fairly consistent volume of air.

Assessing acid–base balance

Steps to assess acid–base balance:
- First, assess on which side of the normal range the pH falls and determine if it is acidemia, alkalemia, or normal
- Second, look at the partial pressure of carbon dioxide ($PaCO_2$) and determine if it is normal, high (acidemia), or low (alkalemia). The $PaCO_2$ indicates involvement of the respiratory system and can be altered by the respiratory rate of the patient
- Third, assess the metabolic component of the blood gas values by looking at the serum bicarbonate (HCO_3^-). If it is high, it is showing more base than if it is low and more acidic in nature
- Fourth, determine if either the $PaCO_2$ or the HCO_3^- can explain the pH. If the pH is normal when the other values are not, then the pH is being compensated

Arterial blood gas sample

An arterial blood gas sample should be drawn, using a heparinized and vented syringe. This allows for the sample to rise in the syringe by the arterial pressure. Heparin is critical to prevent coagulation of the sample both while in the syringe and while moving through the blood gas analyzer. Pressure must be applied to the artery for 5 minutes after drawing a sample. If a collected sample remains at room temperature for more than 15 minutes, changes will occur in the partial pressures of oxygen (PaO_2) and carbon dioxide ($PaCO_2$) and pH. These changes are from natural metabolism occurring within the blood. The best way to slow down the metabolism for delayed analysis is to decrease the temperature of a sample collected in a glass syringe by placing it in an ice bath. Blood gas samples obtained in plastic syringes should not be placed in ice baths because after 15 minutes the PaO_2 can rise as much as 20 mm Hg, and this artificial reading can effect treatment. Ice baths may alter electrolyte readings.

Point of care units

Point-of-care units used to analyze arterial blood gas (ABG) samples are small and portable, making them ideal for use at the patient bedside. ABG analysis can be taken out of the lab and placed directly into the field where the patient need is greatest. Some point of care units are attached to arterial lines, and lab results can be obtained in 60 seconds or less. Their use drastically shortens the time required for critical results to be delivered to the physician and eases demands on the laboratory. Since the units are compact, they use disposable electrode cassettes, which are tested before each use. Calibration and quality control are included in the electrode cassette. However, the equipment is expensive so it is most cost-effective when multiple readings are required.

ABGs

Arterial blood gases (ABGs) are monitored to assess effectiveness of oxygenation, ventilation, and acid–base status, and to determine oxygen flow rates. Partial pressure of a gas is that exerted by each gas in a mixture of gases, proportional to its concentration, based on total atmospheric pressure of 760 mm Hg at sea level. Normal values include:
- Acidity/alkalinity (pH): 7.35–7.45. The critical value of serum pH is 7.20 or less, the point at which adverse effects occur. Patients who are heavily sedated and not compensating with respirations may develop decreased serum bicarbonate (HCO_3^-) and acidemic pH
- Partial pressure of carbon dioxide ($PaCO_2$): 35–45 mm Hg
- Partial pressure of oxygen (PaO_2): 80 mg Hg or more
- HCO_3^- concentration: 22–26 mEq/L

- Oxygen saturation: 95% or more

The relationship between these elements, particularly the $PaCO_2$ and the PaO_2, indicates respiratory status. For example, a $PaCO_2$ over 55 mm Hg and a PaO_2 less than 60 mm Hg in a patient previously in good health indicates respiratory failure. There are many issues to consider. Ventilator management may require a higher $PaCO_2$ to prevent barotrauma and a lower PaO_2 to reduce oxygen toxicity.

Respiratory acidosis

Respiratory acidosis is precipitated by inadequate ventilation of alveoli, interfering with gaseous exchange so that carbon dioxide increases and oxygen decreases, causing excess carbonic acid (H_2CO_3) levels. The body maintains a normal pH by balancing bicarbonate (HCO_3^-) [renal] with partial pressure of carbon dioxide ($PaCO_2$) [pulmonary] in a 20:1 ratio. If the pH alters, the system (renal or pulmonary) that is not causing the problem compensates. Respiratory acidosis after cardiac surgery is commonly related to central respiratory depression related to cardiac arrest, obesity, drugs (e.g., opiates, sedatives, anesthesia, neuromuscular blocking agents), pulmonary issues (e.g., pulmonary edema or embolism, acute respiratory distress syndrome, aspiration, airway obstruction, pneumothorax, atelectasis, restrictive lung disease, asthma, bronchospasm), increased production of carbon dioxide from shivering or sepsis, hypoventilation, inadequate mechanical ventilation, or ventilation/perfusion ratio.
- Acute: Increased $PaCO_2$ with decreased pH caused by sudden decrease in ventilation
- Chronic: Increased $PaCO_2$ with normal pH and serum HCO_3^- over 30 mm Hg with renal compensation

Arterial blood gas values in respiratory acidosis are as follows:

- pH less than 7.35
- PaCO$_2$ more than 42 mm Hg
- Increased H$_2$CO$_3$

Acute respiratory acidosis

Symptoms	Treatment
Acute respiratory acidosis: Increased heart rate Tachypnea Hypertension Confusion and pressure in head related to cerebrovascular vasodilation, especially if partial pressure of carbon dioxide (PaCO$_2$ more than 60 mm Hg Increased intracranial pressure with papilledema Ventricular fibrillation Hyperkalemia	Improving ventilation; careful use of mechanical ventilation Medications as indicated (depending on cause): bronchodilatorsanticoagulation therapy, diuretics, and antibiotics Pulmonary hygiene

Respiratory alkalosis

Respiratory alkalosis results from hyperventilation, during which extra carbon dioxide is excreted, causing a decrease in carbonic acid (H$_2$CO$_3$) concentration in the plasma. In the cardiac surgery patient, acute respiratory alkalosis may be triggered by hypoventilation related to anxiety or pain; increased demand for oxygen with fever, bacteremia (especially Gram-negative), and sepsis; pulmonary disorders, such as pneumonia, pulmonary edema or embolism; and ventilation/perfusion mismatch. Other causes include incorrect ventilator settings and respiratory stimulants. Chronic respiratory alkalosis may result from chronic hepatic insufficiency, cerebral tumors, and chronic hypocapnia.

Respiratory alkalosis

Characteristics	Decreased partial pressure of carbon dioxide (PaCO$_2$). Normal or decreased serum bicarbonate (HCO$_3^-$) as kidneys conserve hydrogen and excrete HCO$_3^-$ Increased pH
Symptoms	Vasoconstriction with decreased cerebral blood flow, resulting in lightheadedness, alterations in mentation, and unconsciousness Numbness and tingling Tinnitus Tachycardia and dysrhythmias
Treatment	Identifying and treating underlying cause. If respiratory alkalosis is related to anxiety, breathing in a paper bag may increase carbon dioxide level. Some people may require sedation. Arterial blood gas values in respiratory alkalosis: <ul><li>pH over 7.45</li><li>PaCO$_2$ less than 38 mm Hg</li><li>Decreased H$_2$CO$_3$</li></ul>

Metabolic acidosis

Metabolic acidosis is a deficit in base bicarbonate (HCO$_3^-$) and occurs when an acid other than carbonic acid (e.g., ketoacid from diabetic ketoacidosis [DKA], lactic acid from shock) builds up in the body or with loss of HCO$_3^-$ from body (diarrhea) fluids. The compensatory mechanism is increased carbon dioxide excretion through the lungs with Kussmaul respirations and increased renal excretion. Metabolic acidosis in cardiac surgery patients is associated with decreased cardiac output and cardiac function, inadequate systemic and peripheral perfusion, hypotension, hypovolemia, and vasoconstriction (related to hypothermia). Other causes include sepsis, renal failure, renal tubular acidosis, DKA, ischemia, and anaerobic metabolism. Symptoms include drowsiness, confusion, headache, coma, hypotension, arrhythmias (related to compensatory hyperkalemia), peripheral vasodilation, nausea, vomiting, diarrhea, and

deep, rapid respirations. Arterial blood gas values are as follows:
- Increased anion gap (most common)
- Carbonic acid less than 22 mEq/L (decrease a cardinal sign)
- pH less than 7.35
- Decreased partial pressure of carbon dioxide

Treatment includes eliminating excess chloride, HCO_3^- if pH is less than 7.1, and serum HCO_3^- is less than 10 mEq/L. Serum potassium must be monitored during treatment as hypokalemia may occur

Metabolic alkalosis

Metabolic alkalosis occurs with either a loss of base acid (e.g., from vomiting or nasogastric [NG] tube) or a gain in bicarbonate (HCO_3^-). As a compensatory mechanism, the respiratory rate decreases to increase partial pressure of carbon dioxide ($PaCO_2$), and renal excretion of HCO_3^- increases. In cardiac surgery patients, hypokalemia, hypochloremia, excess diuretics (especially thiazides), adrenal disorders, NG suctioning, vomiting, and multiple transfusions of citrated blood products are seen. Hypokalemia and hypocalcemia are commonly found with metabolic alkalosis and must be treated. Symptoms predominately relate to hypocalcemia and can include tingling, hypertonic muscles, and dizziness. Other symptoms include depressed respirations, atrial tachycardia, and ventricular dysrhythmias. Skin turgor is often poor. Arterial blood gas values are as follows:
- pH over 7.45
- Carbonic acid more than 26 mEq/L
- Increased $PaCO_2$

Treatment includes restoring fluid balance and identifying and treating the underlying cause. Potassium chloride or sodium chloride is the primary treatment, depending on the potassium level. Proton pump inhibitors are given with NG suctioning, and doses of loop diuretics and thiazides are reduced. In patients with marked diuresis and loss of potassium, acetazolamide or hydrochloric acid may be administered.

Metabolic and respiratory acidosis comparison

Pathophysiology and laboratory

Factors	Metabolic	Respiratory
Pathophysiology	Increase in fixed acid and inability to excrete acid or loss of base, with compensatory increase of carbon dioxide excretion by lungs	Hypoventilation and carbon dioxide retention, with renal compensatory retention of bicarbonate (HCO_3^-) and increased excretion of hydrogen
Laboratory	Decreased serum pH and partial pressure of carbon dioxide ($PaCO_2$) normal if uncompensated and decreased if compensated; decreased HCO_3^-; and urine pH less than 6 if compensated	Decreased serum pH and increased $PaCO_2$; increased HCO_3^- if compensated and normal if uncompensated; and urine pH less than 6 if compensated
Pathophysiology	Decreased strong acid or increased base, with compensatory carbon dioxide retention by lungs	Hyperventilation and increased excretion of carbon dioxide with compensatory bicarbonate (HCO_3^-) excretion by kidneys
Laboratory	Increased serum pH; partial pressure of carbon dioxide ($PaCO_2$) normal if uncompensated and increased if compensated; increased HCO_3^-; and urine pH more than 6 if compensated	Increased serum pH; decreased $PaCO_2$; HCO_3^- normal if uncompensated and decreased if compensated; and urine pH more than 6 if compensated

Symptoms

Factors	Metabolic	Respiratory
Symptoms	Neuromuscular: drowsiness, confusion headache, and coma Cardiac: decreased blood pressure (BP), arrhythmias, and flushed skin Gastrointestinal: nausea, vomiting, abdominal pain, and diarrhea Respiratory: deep inspired tachypnea	Neuromuscular: drowsiness, dizziness, headache, coma, disorientation, and seizures Cardiac: flushed skin, ventricular fibrillation, and decreased BP Gastrointestinal: absent Respiratory: hypoventilation with hypoxia
Symptoms	Neuromuscular: dizziness, confusion, nervousness, anxiety, tremors, muscle cramping, tetany, tingling, and seizures Cardiac: tachycardia and arrhythmias Gastrointestinal: nausea, vomiting, and anorexia. Respiratory: compensatory hypoventilation	Neuromuscular: light-headed, confused, and lethargic Cardiac: tachycardia and arrhythmias Gastrointestinal: epigastric pain, nausea, and vomiting Respiratory: hyperventilation

Causes

Factors	Metabolic	Respiratory
Causes	Diabetic ketoacidosis, lactic acidosis, diarrhea, starvation, renal failure, shock, and renal tubular acidosis	Chronic obstructive pulmonary disease, overdose of sedative or barbiturate, obesity, severe pneumonia/atelectasis, muscle weakness (Guillain-Barré), and mechanical hypoventilation
Causes	Excessive vomiting, gastric suctioning, diuretics, potassium deficit, and excessive mineralocorticoids and serum bicarbonate intake.	Hyperventilation associated with hypoxia, pulmonary embolus, exercise, anxiety, pain, and fever; encephalopathy, septicemia, brain injury, salicylate overdose, and mechanical hyperventilation

Chronic respiratory acidosis

Symptoms	Treatment
Chronic respiratory acidosis: Symptoms may be subtler with chronic respiratory acidosis because of the compensatory mechanisms. If the $PaCO_2$ remains over 50 mm Hg for long periods, the respiratory center becomes increasingly insensitive to the carbon dioxide as a respiratory stimulus, replaced by hypoxemia, so supplemental oxygen administration should	Improving ventilation; careful use of mechanical ventilation Medications as indicated (depending on cause): bronchodilatorsanticoagulation therapy, diuretics, and antibiotics Pulmonary hygiene

Hyperglycemia and Hypoglycemia Management

Hyperglycemia management

Both nondiabetics and diabetics may exhibit hyperglycemia because of hormonal stress, causing insulin resistance, total parenteral nutrition, or sepsis and is associated with an increased risk of osmotic diuresis, impaired wound healing, impaired cognitive function, and atrial fibrillation; thus, blood glucose levels must be monitored carefully and maintained at less than 180 mg/dL (usually 110–150 mg/dL) during the first 48 hours postoperatively although stringent methods to keep blood glucose less than 120 mg/dL are contraindicated. Novolin R, fast-acting regular insulin, is used most frequently with a bolus followed by an infusion (100 U/100 mL normal saline). Potassium should be monitored as well and maintained between 4 and 4.5 mEq/L. Patients with preexisting diabetes type 1 may receive a low dose (about 50% of normal dose) of intermediate or long-acting insulin supplemented with regular insulin. Patients with diabetes type 2 may require regular insulin after surgery and should resume oral medications when able to eat a normal diet. Note that hypoglycemia and diabetic ketoacidosis rarely occur after cardiac surgery.

Glycemic disorders

Insulin is used to metabolize glucose after cardiac surgery to control hyperglycemia induced by hormonal stress and insulin resistance. Duration of action may vary, according to the individual's metabolism, intake, and level of activity. The types of insulin commonly used for hyperglycemia after cardiac surgery include the following:

- Humalog (Lispro H) is a fast-acting, short-duration insulin that acts within 5–15 minutes, peaks between 45–90 minutes, and lasts 3–4 hours

- Novolog (Aspart) is a fast-acting, short-duration insulin that acts within 5–10 minutes, peaks in 1–3 hours, and lasts 3–5 hours
- Regular (R) is a relatively fast-acting insulin that acts within 30 minutes, peaks in 2–5 hours, and lasts 5–8 hours
- NPH (N) is an intermediate-acting insulin that acts in 1–3 hours, peaks at 6–12 hours (Humulin N) or 4–12 hours (Novolin N), and lasts 16–24 hours
- Lantus (Glargine) is a long-acting insulin that acts in 1 hour and lasts 24 hours with no peak

Acute hypoglycemia management

Acute hypoglycemia (hyperinsulinism) results from the use of insulin to control hyperglycemia after cardiac surgery. Hyperinsulinism can cause damage to the central nervous system and cardiopulmonary system, interfering with brain function and causing neurological impairment. Causes include the following:

- Severe infections, such as Gram-negative sepsis and endotoxic shock
- Too much insulin for body needs
- Too little food

Symptoms	Treatment
Blood glucose less than 50–60 mg/dL Central nervous system: seizures, altered consciousness, lethargy, poor feeding with vomiting, myoclonus, respiratory distress, diaphoresis, hypothermia, and cyanosis Adrenergic system: diaphoresis, tremor, tachycardia, palpitation, hunger, and anxiety	Treatment depends on the underlying cause and includes the following: Glucose/glucagon administration to elevate blood glucose levels Diazoxide (Hyperstat) to inhibit release of insulin Somatostatin (Sandostatin) to suppress insulin production Careful monitoring

Management of Recovery from Anesthesia

Emergence from anesthesia

Emergence from anesthesia must be carefully managed and varies, depending on the type of anesthetic agents used. If muscle relaxants are used to paralyze muscles during surgery, then the effects must be reversed before emergence and removal of ventilation so that the patient can breathe independently. Administration of the muscle relaxant is discontinued, and a reversing agent, such as an anticholinesterase, may be used. With general anesthesia, patients may be able to follow verbal directions soon after the anesthetic agent is discontinued, and the intubation tube can be removed unless the patient is to be continued on ventilation. In that case, the patient may be transferred to the postanesthesia unit before awakening. Patients may have some persistent difficulty thinking after emergence because of the lasting effects of some anesthetic agents. Because of respiratory depression, a common side effect of most anesthetic agents, careful monitoring of oxygen saturation and ventilation must be done during the recovery period, and supplemental oxygen is provided to improve oxygen saturation.

Airway devices

ETTS
Endotracheal/tracheal tubes (ETTs) are usually made of radiopaque polyvinyl chloride plastic that is pliable and able to mold to the shape of the airway. They are used to deliver anesthetic gases and oxygen directly to the trachea. ETTs are sized according to internal diameter. The tip ends are beveled, and Murphy tracheal tubes have an opening (Murphy eye) at the distal end to reduce the chance of occlusion. A large size increases airflow but can cause more trauma than small sizes. Adult ETTs usually have an inflatable cuff to affect a tracheal seal, which allows positive pressure ventilation and prevents aspiration. Cuffs may be high pressure (low volume), which can cause ischemia and mucosal trauma, and are not suitable for long anesthesia or ventilation. Low-pressure (high volume) cuffs are used more frequently and cause less trauma, but they increase the risk of sore throat, aspiration, and spontaneous extubation.

TEE

Transesophageal echocardiography (TEE) is commonly used for monitoring during cardiac surgery, providing information about cardiac function and anatomy. TEE uses ultrasound waves from a piezoelectric crystal. These waves penetrate tissue and bounce back, creating a display. Multiple views can be obtained from different areas of the esophagus. M-mode gives a one-dimensional view and is useful for velocity. B-mode is two-dimensional and provides a cross section that shows cardiac performance. Live three-dimensional echocardiography displays images in vector format and allows better visualization and assessment. Pulsed-wave Doppler and continuous-wave Doppler measure velocity. TEE is used most commonly to assess ventricular function, myocardial ischemia, stroke volume (ejection fraction), function of valves (aortic and mitral), residual intracardiac air, fluid volume, cardiac structures, and abnormalities (tamponade and pericarditis). TEE helps to monitor the effects of anesthesia on cardiac function and may be used postoperatively to evaluate potential problems, such as low cardiac output, marked hypotension, or cardiac tamponade.

Transfer from OR to ICU

During transfer from the operating room to the intensive care unit (ICU), patients are usually ventilated with an Ambu bag during transfer, and medications are maintained with battery-powered infusion pumps. The patient must be monitored carefully for changes in hemodynamic status and electrocardiogram (ECG) tracings during transfer, and ECG and monitoring devices are transferred and checked one at a time. The endotracheal tube should be attached to the bedside ventilator, and all settings must be verified. Thoracic drainage tubes should be attached to suction. Common problems encountered include hypotension and inaccurate ECG tracings. Hypotension (systolic < 90 mm Hg or mean < 60 mm Hg) is usually associated with hypovolemia or stopping medications. All dosages of medications and infusion must be checked, and all tubes and attachments must be checked for kinks or occlusions. Chest tubes must be examined for evidence of hemorrhage. A portable chest x-ray should be done in the operating room or on admission to the ICU to evaluate the position of tubes and catheters and to note the width of the mediastinum or evidence of a pneumothorax, atelectasis, pleural effusion, or fluid overload.

Hypotension management

Inaccurate zeroing of the transducer may result in hypotension in the immediate postoperative period, so low blood pressure (BP) should be verified before initiating treatment. To determine if the tracing is dampened:

- Check bilateral breath sounds during manual ventilation.
- Take an auscultatory/occlusive BP reading.
- Monitor all medications and dosages, and make sure infusion rates are set properly.
- Note signs of excessive mediastinal bleeding.
- Check cardiac filling pressures, and make sure that all transducers are placed correctly and that all monitors are calibrated. (Filling pressures may be inaccurate in the immediate postoperative period.) Low-filling pressures can indicate hypovolemia, and high-filling pressures can indicate myocardial dysfunction.

- Treat confirmed hypotension with fluid resuscitation. If there is no response, administer calcium chloride, 500 mg, intravenously. Vasoactive drugs may be initiated or dosages altered.
- If there is no response to previous actions and BP remains life-threateningly low, then the patient may be on the verge of cardiac arrest and may need to have resternotomy.

Blood warmers

Rapid infusions of cold blood may cause cardiac dysrhythmias. Blood warmers are used to warm blood to approximately 32°C–38°C. Indications for blood warmers include the following:

- Prevention of or increase in hypothermia
- Blood flow rate of more than 100 mL/min (adult)
- Patient evidence of significant cold agglutinins
- Rapid infusion, using central lines

Blood warmers must be approved by the Food and Drug Administration. The American Association of Blood Bank standards require that blood be attached to a warmer for no more than 4 hours. Overheating blood (> 42°C) may cause hemolysis, so blood warmers must have temperature controls with a visible thermometer and an online monitor that includes an audible alarm system. There are a number of different types of blood warming devices:

- Water baths
- Warming plates
- Heat exchangers with heated chambers through which blood flows in a separate chamber
- Mixing devices that combine equal volumes of normal saline (70°C) and red blood cells (4°C)

Delayed emergence

Delayed emergence (failure to emerge for 30–60 minutes after anesthesia ends) is more common in the elderly because of the slowed metabolism of anesthetic agents, but it may have a variety of causes, such as drug overdose during surgery and overdose related to preinduction use of drugs or alcohol that potentiates intraoperative drugs. In this case, naloxone or flumazenil may be indicated if opioids or benzodiazepines are implicated but should be avoided unless absolutely necessary. Physostigmine may also be used to reverse the effects of some anesthetic agents. Hypothermia may also cause delay in emergence, especially core temperatures of less than 33°C and may require forced-air warming blankets to increase the temperature. Other metabolic conditions, such as hypoglycemia or hyperglycemia may also affect emergence. Patients suffering from delayed emergence must be evaluated for perioperative stroke, especially after neurological, cardiovascular, or cerebrovascular surgery. Metabolic disturbances may also delay emergence.

PONV

Postoperative nausea and vomiting (PONV) varies with the type of anesthetic agent used. It occurs in about 20%–30% of postanesthesia patients and may be delayed up to 24 hours. Inhalational agents have a higher incidence of PONV than intravenous, and the incidence is lower with epidural or subarachnoid administration, although it may indicate the onset of hypotension. PONV correlates with the duration of surgery, with longer surgeries causing increased PONV. If high doses of narcotics, propofol, or nitrous oxide are used, PONV is often a problem. PONV is most common in young women and also relates to menstruation. It is also increased in patients with a history of smoking or motion sickness. PONV may be associated with postoperative pain, so managing pain is an important factor in preventing PONV.

Postanesthetic respiratory complications

Respiratory complications are most common in the postanesthesia period, so monitoring oxygen levels is critical to preventing hypoxemia. Patients who are extubated in the operating room must be carefully monitored.

Airway obstruction may be partial or total. Partial obstruction is indicated by sonorous or wheezing respirations, and total obstruction is indicated by the absence of breath sounds. Treatment includes supplemental oxygen, airway insertion, repositioning (jaw thrust), or succinylcholine and positive-pressure ventilation for laryngospasm. If edema of the glottis is causing obstruction, intravenous corticosteroids may be used.

Hypoventilation (partial pressure of carbon dioxide > 45 mm Hg) is often mild but may cause respiratory acidosis. It is usually related to depression caused by anesthetic agents. A number of factors may slow emergence (e.g., hypothermia, overdose, metabolism) and cause hypoventilation. Hypoventilation may also be related to splinting because of pain, requiring additional pain management.

Hypoxemia (mild is a partial pressure of oxygen of 50–60 mm Hg) is usually related to hypoventilation or increased right-to-left shunting and is usually treated with supplementary oxygen (30%–60%) with or without positive airway pressure.

Analgesia and sedation

Patients usually are anesthetized and intubated upon admission to the intensive care unit after surgery but may require postoperative analgesia and sedation. With early extubation, a short-acting agent, such as propofol, is usually used, but patients may experience pain and require additional medication within a few hours. Before discontinuation of propofol, nonsteroidal anti-inflammatory drugs may be administered. These include ketorolac, 30 mg intravenously (IV) [preferred because it inhibits platelet aggregation]; indomethacin, 50 mg rectally; or diclofenac, 75 mg rectally. Morphine sulfate may be given by IV infusion (0.02 mg/kg/hr for patients < 65 years of age and 0.01 mg/kg/hr for those > 65 years of age). If the patient becomes agitated with a reduction in propofol, dexmedetomidine may improve weaning from ventilation, although propofol and fentanyl can be used for a number of days if extubation is delayed. Breakthrough pain is controlled with boluses of morphine or ketorolac or with patient-controlled anesthesia (PCA) on the first postoperative day. Morphine, fentanyl, or remifentanil are used with PCA.

Practice Test

Practice Test Questions

1. An obese 70-year-old man with a history of atrial fibrillation is recovering from open-heart surgery for aortic valve replacement. To decrease the risk of developing postoperative atrial fibrillation, which of the following medications is most commonly administered for prophylaxis?
    a. Metoprolol or atenolol
    b. Amiodarone
    c. Sotalol
    d. Magnesium sulfate

2. Which of the following conditions is most likely to put patients at risk for developing a postoperative embolic stroke?
    a. Ascending aortic manipulation
    b. Ventricular fibrillation
    c. Coronary artery atherosclerosis
    d. Renal disease

3. Isoproterenol is indicated for which of the following clinical situations?
    a. Low cardiac output with decreased systemic vascular resistance and mild hypotension
    b. Decreased systemic vascular resistance with hypotension and adequate cardiac output
    c. Right ventricular dysfunction with increased pulmonary vascular resistance
    d. Improvement of donor heart function in brain-dead patients

4. The primary indications for renal replacement therapy for acute renal failure are
    a. hypovolemia, metabolic alkalosis, and hypokalemia.
    b. initial signs of oliguria.
    c. increasing levels of serum creatinine.
    d. fluid overload, metabolic acidosis, and hyperkalemia.

5. In which of the following surgical procedures is pulmonary valve stenosis treated by making a midsternal incision and a small hole into the heart through which the surgeon inserts a finger or dilator to repair the valve without direct visualization?
    a. Open commissurotomy
    b. Closed surgical valvuloplasty
    c. Annuloplasty
    d. Leaflet repair

6. Which of the following antidysrhythmic drugs is most likely to result in bradycardia, hypotension, heart failure, PR prolongation, and constipation?
    a. Lidocaine
    b. Ibutilide
    c. Amiodarone
    d. Diltiazem

7. A patient is recovering from open-heart surgery and cardiopulmonary bypass for valvuloplasty. She exhibits increased heart rate, arterial hypotension, decreased pulmonary artery wedge pressure, and decreased central venous pressure. These symptoms are consistent with
    a. hypervolemia.
    b. hypovolemia.
    c. cardiac tamponade.
    d. hyperthermia.

8. A patient recovering from mitral valve repair and cardiopulmonary bypass has chest tubes placed in the mediastinum and right pleural cavity with suction set at –20 cm H₂O. Bloody discharge in the first 4 hours was 120 mL, but when the patient is turned to the side, 70 mL of dark red blood drains immediately through the chest tube, and then discharge slows. Hemodynamic status is currently stable. The most likely cause of the increased discharge is
    a. acute onset of bleeding.
    b. repositioning of the chest tube.
    c. pooling of blood.
    d. inadequate protamine dosing.

9. A patient who had undergone coronary artery bypass grafting surgery had 180 mL of bloody discharge through the chest tube in the first 4 hours after surgery, but drainage abruptly slowed. Signs and symptoms include hypotension, tachycardia, muffled heart sounds, increased central venous pressure, and decreased urinary output. Pulsus paradoxus is evident. Chest x-ray shows no enlargement of the cardiac silhouette or widening of the mediastinum. The most likely diagnosis is
    a. cardiac tamponade.
    b. hypovolemia.
    c. ventricular dysfunction.
    d. cardiac failure.

10. Which of the following allergies places a patient at risk for anaphylactic reaction to protamine?
    a. Milk products
    b. Tree nuts
    c. Soy
    d. Fish products

11. A patient received abciximab (ReoPro) to prevent cardiac ischemia while undergoing percutaneous cardiac intervention. Abciximab-induced coagulopathy can occur if abciximab is administered with
    a. aspirin.
    b. weight-adjusted, low-dose heparin.
    c. non–weight-adjusted, long-acting heparin.
    d. β-blockers.

12. Abnormal pulsus paradoxus is characterized by systolic blood pressure that is
    a. 5 mm Hg or less higher during inhalation than exhalation.
    b. 5 mm Hg or less lower during inhalation than exhalation.
    c. more than 10 mm Hg higher during inhalation than exhalation.
    d. more than 10 mm Hg lower during inhalation than exhalation.

13. A postoperative patient has increased bleeding from the chest tube and has developed widespread petechiae and gastrointestinal bleeding over the last 3 hours. Signs and symptoms include the following:

- Blood pressure: 80/40 mm Hg
- Heart rate: 120 bpm
- Respirations: 32 breaths/min
- Temperature: 38.6°C
- Prothrombin time: 6 seconds
- Fibrinogen: 0.8 mg/dL
- Platelet count: 50,000/mm³

The patient is exhibiting increasing signs of shock. The most likely cause of these signs is
    a. acute liver failure.
    b. disseminated intravascular coagulopathy.
    c. hemolytic uremic syndrome.
    d. heparin-induced thrombocytopenia.

14. A patient who has undergone coronary artery bypass grafting surgery with a left internal thoracic artery graft had topical hypothermia of the heart and phrenic nerve during surgery. Following cardiac surgery, especially in which there is topical hypothermia of the heart and phrenic nerve, the patient is at increased risk for
    a. left lower lobe atelectasis.
    b. right lower lobe atelectasis.
    c. cardiac ischemia.
    d. stroke.

15. A patient exhibits increasing confusion and weakness with ascending paralysis and changes in the electrocardiogram following open-heart surgery and cardiopulmonary bypass. Changes include the following:

- ST depression with peaked T waves
- Prolonged PR interval with some loss of P waves and small R waves
- QRS widening

These changes are consistent with which of the following?
    a. Hypokalemia
    b. Hyperkalemia
    c. Hypocalcemia
    d. Hypercalcemia

16. Weaning patients from mechanical ventilation in the initial postoperative period includes which of the following criteria?
    a. Core temperature of 35.2°C
    b. Heart rate of 124 bpm
    c. Slight arrhythmia
    d. Chest tube drainage of 40 mL/hr

17. Using the RIFLE criteria for classifying increasing renal failure, a patient with a 200% increase of serum creatinine, a 50% or more decrease in the glomerular filtration rate, and a urine output of less than 0.5 mL/kg/hr over 12 hours is classified as which of the following?
   a. Risk
   b. Injury
   c. Failure
   d. Loss

18. An elderly patient who had on-pump coronary artery bypass grafting surgery is experiencing sudden onset of confusion, hallucinations, language and memory disturbance, and a reduced ability to focus or sustain attention. Symptoms fluctuate with periods of clarity. The most likely diagnosis is
   a. transient ischemic episode.
   b. stroke.
   c. delirium.
   d. hypoxic-ischemic encephalopathy.

19. A patient who had coronary artery bypass grafting surgery and mitral valve replacement develops postoperative jaundice and low-grade elevations of liver function tests (e.g., alanine aminotransferase, aspartate aminotransferase, bilirubin, alkaline phosphatase). Mental status is unchanged, and blood glucose level is low normal. These symptoms are indicative of
   a. mild hyperbilirubinemia.
   b. hepatic dysfunction.
   c. acute hepatic failure.
   d. chronic hepatic failure.

20. A patient who had coronary artery bypass grafting (CABG) surgery has had persistent postoperative mediastinal bleeding, an elevated partial thromboplastin time, and a hematocrit of 27 mL/dL, but there are no indications of uremia or cardiac tamponade. Which of the following treatment protocols is most likely to reverse these complications of CABG surgery?
   a. Transesophageal echocardiography
   b. Packed red blood cells
   c. Desmopressin, 0.3 μg/kg intravenously (IV)
   d. Protamine, 25 mg IV for two doses

21. Early postoperative blood glucose levels should be maintained at less than which of the following levels to decrease the risk of a wound infection?
   a. 180 mg/dL
   b. 160 mg/dL
   c. 140 mg/dL
   d. 110/mg/dL

22. After removal of a chest tube, a patient complained of retrosternal and neck pain, was dyspneic, and had slight neck edema. Hamman's sign was positive (precordial systolic crepitus). The probable diagnosis is
   a. pneumothorax.
   b. cardiac tamponade.
   c. pneumomediastinum.
   d. pneumopericardium.

23. A patient who just had surgery to replace an aortic valve developed postoperative dyspnea, dry nonproductive cough, chest pain, and orthopnea but remained hemodynamically stable with only a slight temperature elevation. Chest x-ray showed an area of opacity in the left lower lobe. The most likely diagnosis is
   a. hemothorax.
   b. pleural effusion.
   c. pneumothorax.
   d. pneumonia.

24. The postoperative pulmonary artery pressure should be maintained at
   a. less than 10 mm Hg.
   b. less than 15 mm Hg.
   c. more than 25 mm Hg.
   d. less than 25 mm Hg.

25. A 48-year old man with Marfan's syndrome had a surgical repair of a thoracic aortic aneurysm. A potential complication specific to thoracic repair that does not usually occur with other types of aortic aneurysms is
   a. stroke.
   b. hemorrhage.
   c. spinal cord injury with paralysis.
   d. dysrhythmias.

26. The surgical procedure that requires about a 10-cm incision in the mid chest rather than midsternally and is done without cardiopulmonary bypass is
   a. port access coronary artery bypass graft.
   b. minimally invasive direct coronary artery bypass.
   c. transmyocardial laser revascularization.
   d. directional coronary atherectomy.

27. Patients with valve replacements requiring long-term anticoagulation with warfarin usually have individualized target international normalized ratios between
   a. 4 and 5.
   b. 3 and 4.
   c. 1 and 2.
   d. 2 and 3.5.

28. The primary postoperative method of providing core warming after cardiopulmonary bypass is with
   a. peripheral vasoconstriction.
   b. vasodilation.
   c. heated intravenous fluids.
   d. heated humidifiers in a ventilator circuit.

29. For patients with mitral valve surgery, the maze procedure (i.e., a series of incisions in the left atrium) is indicated for the treatment of
   a. ventricular tachycardia.
   b. atrial fibrillation.
   c. hypertrophic obstructive cardiomyopathy.
   d. heart failure.

Copyright © Mometrix Media. You have been licensed one copy of this document for personal use only.
Any other reproduction or redistribution is strictly prohibited. All rights reserved.

30. A patient had on-pump coronary artery bypass grafting surgery and has both atrial and ventricular pacing wires. Which of the following pacing is indicated for sinus bradycardia with normal atrioventricular (AV) conduction?
   a. Atrial pacing
   b. AV sequential pacing
   c. Bi-ventricular pacing
   d. VVI pacing

31. Postoperative administration of aspirin after coronary artery bypass grafting surgery is specifically indicated to prevent occlusion of
   a. internal thoracic artery grafts.
   b. gastroepiploic artery grafts.
   c. saphenous vein grafts.
   d. radial artery grafts.

32. A patient had an intra-aortic balloon pump placed during surgery for left ventricular failure. When the patient stabilizes, the balloon is removed percutaneously. Initial pressure is applied
   a. directly over the insertion site.
   b. proximal to the insertion site.
   c. directly over the skin puncture site.
   d. distal to the insertion site.

33. Side effects of dobutamine include
   a. premature ventricular contractions.
   b. bradycardia.
   c. decreased systolic blood pressure.
   d. hyperkalemia.

34. The critical value for serum pH with metabolic acidosis is
   a. 7.40.
   b. 7.30.
   c. more than 7.60.
   d. less than 7.20.

35. Which of the following signs and symptoms is characteristic of a superficial mediastinal wound infection?
   a. Purulent discharge
   b. Unstable sternum
   c. Leukocytosis
   d. Fever and chills

36. A postoperative patient is evaluated for extubation in the intensive care unit. Which of the following findings regarding respiratory mechanics meets extubation criteria?
   a. Vital capacity: 8 mL/kg
   b. Negative inspiratory force: 23 cm H2O
   c. Spontaneous respiratory rate: 28 breaths/min
   d. Tidal volume: 6 mL/kg

37. Which of the following is an indication of failure during weaning from the ventilator?
    a. Systolic blood pressure increases from 110 mm Hg to 120 mm Hg.
    b. Respiratory rate increases from 22 breaths/min to 30 breaths/min.
    c. The saturation of oxygen in hemoglobin falls from 94% to 88%.
    d. The partial pressure of oxygen in arterial blood falls from 75 torr to 70 torr.

38. A postoperative patient recovering from open-heart surgery has adequate cardiac function but a continual volume requirement needed to maintain filling pressure. Systolic blood pressure is 70 mm Hg. The patient has already received 2 L of fluid. Which of the following treatments is preferred to improve systemic blood pressure and renal blood flow at this point?
    a. Phenylephrine
    b. Norepinephrine
    c. Furosemide
    d. Hespan

39. Which of the following hourly bleeding rates indicates the need for emergent reopening of the chest?
    a. More than 400 mL/hr for 1 hour
    b. Approximately 300 mL/hr for 1 hour
    c. More than 200 mL/hr for 2–3 hours
    d. More than 150 mL/hr for 4 hours

40. When emergent chest reopening and internal defibrillation are necessary in the intensive care unit (ICU), the primary responsibility of the sterile cardiac ICU nurse is
    a. removing dressings and Steri-strips.
    b. preparing medications and gathering equipment.
    c. ensuring strict sterile technique.
    d. preparing the defibrillator machine.

41. The purpose of diuresis with loop diuretics after extubation in stable patients who had cardiopulmonary bypass is to
    a. promote excretion of excess sodium and fluids.
    b. reverse oliguria.
    c. reduce capillary leaks.
    d. promote vasodilation.

42. Patients with nasogastric tubes inserted during surgery for gastric decompression should receive which of the following medications by instillation during the first 12–24 hours?
    a. H_2-blocker (ranitidine)
    b. Proton-pump inhibitor (omeprazole)
    c. Promotility agent (metoclopramide)
    d. Antiulcer drug (sucralfate)

43. Type I atrial flutter (< 350 bpm) can be terminated by
    a. rapid ventricular pacing.
    b. rapid atrial pacing.
    c. bi-ventricular pacing.
    d. atrioventricular pacing.

44. Which of the following can pose the risk of an electrical current triggering an impulse for those with epicardial pacing wires?
    a. Grounded electric bed
    b. Battery-powered shaver
    c. Carpeting
    d. Humidified room air

45. A patient who receives multiple transfusions with citrated blood products must be monitored closely for
    a. hyponatremia.
    b. hypomagnesemia.
    c. hypokalemia.
    d. hypocalcemia.

46. A cardiopulmonary bypass patient has received β-blockers and opioids for pain and develops sinus bradycardia with a rate of 52 bpm. He is treated with atrial pacing but fails to capture and does not respond adequately to epinephrine. The next most likely treatment is
    a. repeat atrial pacing.
    b. ventricular pacing.
    c. atropine.
    d. transcutaneous pacing.

47. A postoperative patient with significantly increased mediastinal bleeding and a fibrinogen level of 90 mg/dL may be treated with
    a. platelet transfusion.
    b. packed red blood cells.
    c. cryoprecipitate.
    d. fresh frozen plasma.

48. A patient had aortic valve surgery for aortic stenosis. The patient's systolic blood pressure was adequate immediately after surgery but began to increase 12 hours postoperatively. To protect the suture line and reduce the myocardium's oxygen needs, which treatment listed below is indicated?
    a. Vasodilator
    b. β-Blocker
    c. Nesiritide
    d. Furosemide

49. A patient exhibited hypotension, increased pulmonary capillary wedge pressure, decreased cardiac output, and increased systemic vascular resistance. The most appropriate intervention would be
    a. intravenous fluids.
    b. an inotropic agent.
    c. a vasodilator.
    d. a diuretic.

50. A postoperative open-heart surgery patient is receiving thoracic epidural analgesia. The nurse's primary concern is to monitor for
    a. weakness in the lower extremities.
    b. cognitive impairment.
    c. level of pain.
    d. indications of infection.

Answer Explanations

1. A: Low-dose β-blockers, such as metoprolol (25–50 mg twice daily) or atenolol (25 mg daily), are the most common drugs to prevent atrial fibrillation (Afib), decreasing the incidence of Afib by up to 65%. Atrial flutter (> 380 bpm) and Afib (> 380 bpm) occur in up to 30% of patients with open-heart surgery. Risk factors include obesity, chronic obstructive pulmonary disease, valve surgery, and a history of Afib. Amiodarone is sometimes given alone or with β-blockers. Sotalol is an effective negative inotrope but has a number adverse effects. Magnesium sulfate is most effective if administered with β-blockers and with low serum magnesium levels.

2. A: Manipulation of the ascending aorta is a primary risk factor for developing intraoperative or postoperative (most common) embolic strokes. Strokes are also often preceded by a period of atrial fibrillation (Afib), especially if Afib persists for extended periods (48 hours). Care must be exercised with use of heparin as about 30% of infarcts may undergo hemorrhagic conversion. Multiple infarcts of varying sizes may occur following cardiac surgery. Serial computed tomography (CT) scans may be necessary for diagnosis as the initial scan may be negative. Diffusion-weighted magnetic resonance imaging is the most sensitive test, but it may not be available; it may show preoperative undiagnosed infarcts.

3. C: Isoproterenol is indicated for right ventricular dysfunction with increased peripheral vascular resistance (PVR). Isoproterenol increases cardiac output through moderately increased contractility, increases heart rate, and reduces systemic vascular resistance (SVR). Because of the heart's increased need for oxygen, isoproterenol has limited use in patients with coronary artery disease. Dopamine is indicated for low cardiac output with decreased SVR and mild hypotension. Phenylephrine is indicated for decreased SVR with hypotension and adequate cardiac output. Triiodothyronine is indicated for improvement of donor heart function in brain-dead patients.

4. D: The primary indications for renal replacement therapy (RRT) include fluid overload, metabolic acidosis, and hyperkalemia. Other indications include increased confusion, pericarditis, or gastrointestinal bleeding. Increasing oliguria and increasing serum creatinine require further evaluation and may trigger RRT to prevent further kidney damage. Intermittent hemodialysis (administered over 3–4 hours three times a week) and continuous venovenous hemofiltration are commonly used after cardiac surgery for patients requiring RRT. Continuous venovenous systems include slow continuous ultrafiltration, continuous venovenous hemofiltration, and continuous venovenous hemodiafiltration.

5. B: Closed surgical valvuloplasty involves a midsternal incision and a small hole into the heart through which the surgeon inserts a finger or dilator to repair the valve without direct visualization. Open commissurotomy uses cardiopulmonary bypass (CPB) and incision into the heart for direct visualization of the valve. Annuloplasty may be done with CPB and incision into the heart or minimally invasive procedures to repair the valve annulus, the junction of valve leaflets and the heart wall. Leaflet repair is usually done with minimally invasive procedures to repair abnormal leaflets.

6. D: Common adverse effects of calcium channel blockers, such as diltiazem or verapamil, include bradycardia, hypotension, heart failure, PR prolongation, and constipation. Bradycardia results from decreased sinoatrial nodal output and PR prolongations from delays in atrioventricular (AV)

conduction. These drugs may cause marked hypotension and worsening of existing heart failure. Calcium channel blockers, used to treat tachycardia, block the influx of calcium ions across membranes of cardiac and arterial muscle cells, slowing the AV node conduction of impulses into the ventricles, thereby slowing the ventricular rate.

7. B: Hypovolemia is characterized by increased heart rate, arterial hypotension, decreased pulmonary artery wedge pressure, and central venous pressure. Hypovolemia may result from net loss of blood during surgery; surgical hypothermia, resulting in vasodilation as the body warms; and intravenous fluid loss into interstitial spaces because of increased permeability of capillary beds. Hypovolemia is the most common cause of decreased cardiac output in the postsurgical period and is treated with fluid replacement, usually initially crystalloid and then colloid. Packed red blood cells may be required for hemodilution.

8. C: Changing the patient's position may result in increased drainage from the chest tube because of pooling of blood. Acute onset of bleeding is characterized by bright red blood and continuous steady discharge. Dark red blood suggests older blood rather than active bleeding, especially if discharge slows after an initial increase. Chest tube drainage should not exceed 200 mL in 2–6 hours. Excess bleeding may require coagulation studies, repeat chest x-ray to evaluate the width of the mediastinum, and transesophageal echocardiogram if cardiac tamponade suspected.

9. A: Cardiac tamponade is characterized by hypotension, tachycardia, muffled heart sounds, increased central venous pressure, decreased urinary output, and pulsus paradoxus. A sudden decrease in chest tube drainage can occur as fluid and clots accumulate in the pericardial sac, preventing the blood from filling the ventricles and decreasing cardiac output and perfusion of the body, including the kidneys (resulting in decreased urinary output). A change in the cardiac silhouette on x-ray and mediastinal widening is evident in only about 20% of patients with cardiac tamponade.

10. D: Protamine sulfate, a heparin antagonist, is comprised of strongly basic proteins derived from salmon sperm and some other fish, so allergies to fish can put the patient at risk for protamine anaphylactic reaction. Symptoms include the following:
- Sudden onset of weakness, dizziness, and confusion
- Urticaria
- Increased permeability of the vascular system and loss of vascular tone
- Severe hypotension, leading to shock
- Laryngospasm/bronchospasm with obstruction of the airway, causing dyspnea and wheezing
- Nausea, vomiting, and diarrhea
- Seizures, coma, and death

11. C: Abciximab (ReoPro) inhibits the aggregation of platelets and potentiates the action of anticoagulants; it is used with aspirin or weight-adjusted, low-dose heparin. However, its use with non–weight-adjusted, long-acting heparin can cause thrombocytopenia with an increased risk of hemorrhage, especially with readministration of the drug, which can induce the formation of antibodies and an allergic reaction; this reaction is characterized by anaphylaxis and thrombocytopenia, referred to as abciximab-induced coagulopathy. Abciximab can be safely used with most cardiac drugs.

12. D: Pulsus paradoxus is a systolic blood pressure that is markedly lower during inhalation than exhalation. Pulsus paradoxus with a more than 10 mm Hg difference is considered abnormal and is

a common sign of cardiac tamponade. A decrease in blood pressure 10 mm Hg or less during inspiration is a normal finding, but an increased pressure difference may indicate a number of cardiopulmonary complications, including pericardial effusion, pericarditis, pulmonary embolism, cardiogenic shock, chronic obstructive pulmonary disease, asthma, and obstruction of the superior vena cava. Blood pressure should be reevaluated if pulsus paradoxus is found to ensure correct readings.

13. B: Disseminated intravascular coagulation triggers both coagulation and hemorrhage through a complex series of events that includes trauma that causes tissue factor (transmembrane glycoprotein) to enter the circulation and bind with coagulation factors, triggering the coagulation cascade. Clotting and hemorrhage continue at the same time, placing the patient at high risk for death, even with treatment. Symptoms include the following:
- Bleeding from surgical or venous puncture sites
- Evidence of gastrointestinal bleeding with distention and bloody diarrhea
- Hypotension and acute symptoms of shock
- Petechiae and purpura with extensive bleeding into the tissues
- Prolonged prothrombin and partial thromboplastin times
- Decreased platelet counts and fragmented red blood cells
- Decreased fibrinogen

14. A: Direct topical hypothermia (cold cardioplegia) to the heart can damage the left phrenic nerve and cause paresis or paralysis of the diaphragm, resulting in an increased incidence of left lower lobe atelectasis. Harvesting of the internal thoracic artery is also associated with high rates of pleural effusions and atelectasis. Symptoms may be evident in the immediate postoperative period and include splinting, decreased ventilation, decreased oxygen saturation, and increased heart rate. Deep breathing, use of an incentive spirometer, or intermittent positive pressure breathing treatments may all help to prevent atelectasis.

15. B: Hyperkalemia may occur with high levels of potassium in cardioplegia solutions during surgery, low cardiac output, marked tissue ischemia, renal insufficiency, medications (e.g., β-blockers, angiotensin-converting enzyme inhibitors, angiotensin receptor blockers, potassium sparing diuretics), and metabolic/respiratory acidosis. Normal values are 3.5–5.5 mEq/L. Asystolic arrest may occur at levels over 6.5 mEq/L. The primary symptoms relate to the effect on the cardiac muscle:
- Ventricular arrhythmias with increasing changes in the electrocardiogram, leading to cardiac and respiratory arrest
- Weakness with ascending paralysis and hyperreflexia
- Diarrhea
- Increasing confusion

16. D: Chest tube drainage of 40 mL/hr meets the criteria (< 50 mL/hr) for weaning from ventilation in the initial postoperative period. Other criteria include adequate reversal of neuromuscular blockade and an awake state without stimulation. Core temperature should be over 35.5°C. Hemodynamic status should be stable with a cardiac index of over 2.2 L/min/m², systolic blood pressure of 100–140 mm Hg, a heart rate of less than 120 bpm, and no arrhythmias. Blood gases should be stable on ventilation with a pH of 7.30–7.50, partial pressure of carbon dioxide of less than 50 torr, a partial pressure of oxygen in arterial blood over 75 torr, and a fraction of inspired oxygen (FiO_2) of 0.5.

17. B: RIFLE classifications (in order) include risk, injury, failure, loss, and end-stage kidney disease. Risk (most common) includes increased serum creatinine by 150% or decreased glomerular filtration rate (GFR) by 25% or more with urinary output less than 0.5 mL/kg/hr over 6 hours. Injury includes increased serum creatinine by 200% or decreased GFR by 50% or more with urine output less than 0.5 mL/kg/hr over 12 hours. Failure includes increased serum creatinine by 300%, decreased GFR by 75% or more, serum creatinine over 4 mg/dL, or an acute rise in serum creatinine to 0.5 mg/dL or more with urine output less than 0.3 mL/kg/hr over 24 hours. Loss is acute renal failure persisting for 4 weeks or more and end stage kidney disease persisting for 3 months or more.

18. C: Delirium is an acute sudden change in consciousness, characterized by a reduced ability to focus or sustain attention, language and memory disturbance, disorientation, confusion, audiovisual hallucinations, sleep disturbance, and psychomotor activity disorder. Delirium differs from disorders with similar symptoms in that delirium is fluctuating. Delirium may result from drugs, such as anticholinergics, and numerous conditions, including infection, hypoxia, trauma, dementia, depression, vision and hearing loss, surgery, alcoholism, untreated pain, fluid/electrolyte imbalance, and malnutrition. Delirium increases the risks of morbidity and death, especially if untreated.

19. B: Hepatic dysfunction is common after cardiac surgery, especially with prolonged cardiopulmonary bypass and multiple procedures. It is characterized by transient low-grade elevation of liver function tests. About a fourth of patients will develop hyperbilirubinemia and jaundice with bilirubin more than 3 mg/dL, but less than 1% progress to postpump liver failure, which is characterized by coagulopathy, hypoglycemia, renal failure, encephalopathy, and refractory acidosis. Elevated bilirubin by itself is usually benign and self-limiting. Patients must be monitored carefully for coagulopathy during periods of hepatic dysfunction, as the impaired liver may not produce adequate clotting factors.

20. D: Protamine (25 mg intravenously [IV] for two doses) is indicated for postoperative mediastinal bleeding if the partial thromboplastin time is elevated. Although protamine is given at the end of surgery to reverse heparin, a heparin rebound effect may occur after surgery, causing increased bleeding; additional infusions of protamine will reduce this effect. Transesophageal echocardiography is indicated if there are concerns about cardiac tamponade. Packed red blood cells are indicated for a hematocrit of less than 26 mL/dL. Desmopressin (0.3 μg/kg IV) is indicated for uremia or platelet dysfunction related to use of aspirin.

21. A: Blood glucose levels should be maintained at less than 180 mg/dL in the first 48 postoperative hours to reduce the risk of wound infection in both diabetics and nondiabetics. The most commonly used insulin is Novolin R, given by bolus followed by infusion of 100 U/100 mL normal saline. Lowering the blood glucose to less than 120 mg/dL is not recommended. Hyperglycemia may develop after surgery because of increased insulin resistance brought about by a stress response, total parenteral nutrition without an adequate insulin response, and sepsis.

22. C: Retrosternal and neck pain, dyspnea, and slight neck edema indicate pneumomediastinum. Hamman's sign—a precordial rasping sound heard on auscultation during a heartbeat as the heart moves against tissues filled with air—is an indication of both pneumomediastinum and pneumopericardium but is not generally present with pneumothorax or cardiac tamponade. Neck edema occurs with pneumomediastinum. Air leaks can occur from damage to the pleura during

surgery or (less commonly) from obstructed chest tubes. Air leaks usually resolve within a few days but may require reinsertion of a chest tube.

23. B: Pleural effusion is common after cardiac surgery and appears as an opacity on a radiograph. Common indications include dyspnea, dry
nonproductive cough, chest pain, and orthopnea, although small effusions may remain asymptomatic. Hemothorax results in a decreased hematocrit and hemodynamic instability. Small pleural effusions resolve over time, but large pleural effusions may require thoracentesis (often with ultrasound guidance) to drain fluid and relieve dyspnea. Correct positioning of chest tubes during surgery can help reduce the incidence of pleural effusions.

24. D: Positive airway pressure (PAP) should be maintained at less than 25 mm Hg postoperatively. PAP is measured by a catheter usually fed through the right ventricle to the main pulmonary artery:
- Normal PAP is 10–20 mg Hg (mean 15 mm Hg). PAP is usually about 25%–34% the systemic blood pressure rate. Oxygen saturation is usually about 80%.
- Increased PAP may indicate pulmonary obstruction or embolus, left-to-right shunt, left ventricular failure, pulmonary hypertension, mitral stenosis, pneumothorax, lung/alveolar hypoplasia, hyperviscosity of blood, or increased left atrial pressure.
- Decreased PAP may indicate a decrease in intravascular volume, decreased cardiac output, or obstruction of pulmonary blood flow.

25. C: There is a 4% occurrence of paraplegia with thoracic aorta aneurysm because of possible damage to the spinal cord during the procedure. The aneurysms are often asymptomatic but may cause substernal pain, back pain, dyspnea, stridor (from pressure on the trachea), cough, distention of neck veins, and edema of the neck and arms. Rupture usually does not allow time for emergent repair, so identifying and correcting before rupture are essential. Surgery is indicated for aneurysms 5–6 cm or more. Endovascular grafting is now routinely done for aneurysms of the descending thoracic aorta.

26. B: Minimally invasive direct coronary artery bypass applies a bypass graft on the beating heart through a 10-cm incision in the mid chest rather than midsternally, without cardiopulmonary bypass (CPB). Port access coronary artery bypass graft uses a number of small incisions (ports) along with CPB and cardioplegia for a video-assisted repair. Transmyocardial laser revascularization may be done percutaneously or through a surgical procedure. Laser bursts cut 20–40 channels into but not through the myocardium. Directional coronary atherectomy uses a large balloon catheter (inserted femorally) with a window on one side with a rotational cutting piston.

27. D: Target international normalized ratios (INRs) are usually between 2 and 3.5 (with 2.5–3.5 most common for valve replacements), varying somewhat according to risk factors. The critical value is more than 3.5 in patients receiving anticoagulation therapy. INRs should be checked daily for the first week and then two to three times weekly until levels stabilize. Adjustment in dosages should be only every 2–3 days because peak response occurs in 36–48 hours. Many medications affect warfarin dosage, so all medications should be evaluated.

28. A: Peripheral vasoconstriction is often used postoperatively after cardiopulmonary bypass (CPB) to provide core warming. Vasodilators redistribute core heat and may slow core warming, although they increase perfusion. Heated intravenous fluid and humidifiers in the ventilator circuits may treat hypothermia but are usually not effective for increasing core temperatures. During CPB,

systemic hypothermia (32°C–34°C) is used, but the patient should be warmed to about 36°C before leaving the operating room. Because brain temperature may be higher than measurable core temperature, raising the temperature to 37°C may impair neurocognitive functioning.

29. B: The maze procedure (i.e., a series of incisions in the left atrium) is usually done with mitral valve surgery to treat atrial fibrillation as restoring normal sinus rhythm improves long-term survival after cardiac surgery. The maze procedure (cut-and-sew) results in ablation lines around and between the right and left pulmonary veins and an additional line from the inferior box lesion by the right or left inferior pulmonary vein to the mitral valve annulus. The left atrial appendage is removed and an ablation line placed from the appendage base to the left pulmonary veins with the base of the appendage oversewn.

30. A: Sinus bradycardia and junctional rhythm are usually treated with atrial pacing (90 bpm) if there is normal atrioventricular conduction. This pacing is usually sufficient to fill the left ventricle adequately and improve cardiac output. Atrioventricular sequential pacing may result in ventricular dyssynchrony. Bi-ventricular (BiV) pacing with an extra set of leads may be used with moderate-to-severe left ventricular dysfunction (RA-BiV) to improve cardiac output. VVI pacing (i.e., single-wire pacing) is used if the patient shows an inadequate ventricular response to atrial fibrillation.

31. C: Postoperative administration of aspirin is indicated to prevent occlusion of saphenous vein grafts. Aspirin has not been shown to improve patency of arterial grafts. Postoperative aspirin (75–100 mg) should be administered within 24 hours after surgery, usually starting at 6 hours. Although the beneficial effects of aspirin on patency are not evident after a year, ongoing use of aspirin in recommended for all graft recipients to prevent further coronary artery disease.

32. D: When an intra-aortic balloon pump is removed percutaneously, initial pressure is applied distal to the insertion site for a few heartbeats to flush out the wound. Then, pressure is applied slightly proximal to the insertion site as the artery puncture site is slightly cephalad to the skin puncture site. Steady pressure should be maintained for 45 minutes or more without interruption to prevent formation of thrombus. The D-STAT dry hemostatic bandage, which contains bovine thrombin, may be used to improve surface hemostasis.

33. A: Side effects of dobutamine include premature ventricular contractions (occurring in about 5%), increased systolic blood pressure, hypotension, and local reactions. Dobutamine improves cardiac output, treats cardiac decompensation, and lowers blood pressure. It helps the body to use norepinephrine. Dobutamine is used short-term for cardiac decompensation after cardiac surgery as it increases the force of myocardial contractions with minimal effect on heart rate. Dobutamine is contraindicated with hypovolemia and acute myocardial infarction and must be used with caution in patients with diabetes or an allergy to sulfites (most common in patients with asthma).

34. D: The critical value of serum pH is less than 7.20, the point at which adverse effects occur. Patients who are heavily sedated and not compensating with respirations may develop decreased sodium bicarbonate and acidemic pH. Metabolic acidosis may result in decreased contractility and cardiac output with subsequent reduction in blood flow to the liver and kidneys, increased pulmonary vascular resistance, vasoconstriction, arteriolar dilatation, increased arrhythmias, ventricular fibrillation, dyspnea, tachypnea, hyperglycemia, hyperkalemia, increased production of lactate, and increased metabolic demands.

35. A: A superficial mediastinal wound infection is characterized by serous or purulent drainage and local tenderness and erythema. A major incisional infection is characterized by increased purulent discharge, fever, chills, leukocytosis, lethargy, unstable sternum, and pain. Symptoms may vary according to the causative organism. *Staphylococcus aureus* infections usually have a rapid onset of symptoms that occur within the first 10 days. Occult infections—especially common with diabetics—often have delayed symptoms with collections of purulent material but few systemic signs of infection.

36. D: A tidal volume of 6 mL/kg meets extubation criteria in the initial postoperative period. Extubation should be done after the patient meets weaning criteria. Extubation can be done from continuous positive airway pressure (CPAP) or T-piece. Criteria include awake state without stimulation and acceptable respiratory mechanics and blood gases (on ≤ 5 cm CPAP or partial specific volume):
- Tidal volume: more than 5 mL/kg
- Negative inspiratory force: more than 25 cm H_2O.
- Vital capacity: more than 10–15 mL/kg
- Respirations (spontaneous): less than 25 breaths/min
- Partial pressure of oxygen in arterial blood: more than 70 torr (on fraction of inspired oxygen ≤ 0.5)
- Partial pressure of carbon dioxide: less than 48 torr
- pH: 7.32–7.45

37. C: Failure criteria for ventilator weaning includes a decrease in the saturation level of oxygen in hemoglobin (SaO_2) to less than 90%. Other indications of weaning failure include agitation, diaphoresis, increased somnolence, change in systolic blood pressure by more than 20 bpm or more than 160 mm Hg, a heart rate increase or decrease of more than 20% or tachycardia with 120 bpm, a need for vasoactive medications to maintain status, development or worsening of arrhythmias, increased respiratory rate of more than 10 breaths/min or more than 35 breaths/min for a 5-minute period, a partial pressure of oxygen of less than 60 torr (on a fraction of inspired oxygen of 0.5), and a partial pressure of carbon dioxide of more than 50 torr with a pH of less than 7.30.

38. B: Norepinephrine is the drug of choice to improve renal blood flow and increase systolic blood pressure if the patient has already received 1.5–2 L of fluid. While the goal of management is to ensure adequate intravascular volume needed for adequate cardiac output and perfusion, excess fluids can induce renal dysfunction and result in hemodilution, which lowers the hemoglobin and hematocrit and reduces clotting factors, increasing the risk of bleeding. Hespan is a volume expander, but it may cause platelet dysfunction.

39. A: An bleeding rate of more than 400 mL for 1 hour indicates the need for emergent reopening of the chest. Reopening should be considered any time there is a sudden onset of excessive bleeding (> 300 mL/hr) because delay is associated with increased morbidity and death with an increased need for transfusions, hemodynamic instability, and the risk of cardiac arrest. Other indications for emergent reopening of the chest include signs of cardiac tamponade and bleeding criteria:
- More than 300 mL/hr for 2–3 hours
- More than 200 mL/hr for 4 hours

40. C: When the intensive care unit is used as an operating room, a sterile nurse must ensure that strict sterile technique is followed. A nonsterile nurse may remove the dressing and Steri-strips, but

the scrub (usually with povidone iodine poured over the chest) should be done by the sterile nurse. The paddles for the internal defibrillator are maintained in sterile coverings, but the machine is not. During the procedure, one nurse should be responsible for recording details of the procedure, another for administration of medications and fluids, and another (circulator) to get necessary equipment or prepare medications while the sterile nurse assists with sterile procedures.

41. A: Loop diuretics, such as furosemide, are used to promote excretion of excess sodium and fluid, usually after the myocardial function has stabilized, inotropic support is decreased, and the patient is extubated. By this time, usually 6–12 hours after surgery, core temperature should be normal, capillary leaks stopped, and filling pressures stabilized. Diuretics are usually avoided in the first 6 hours after surgery except for the occurrence of marked oliguria or pulmonary edema associated with reduced oxygenation.

42. D: Antiulcer drugs, such as sucralfate, should be instilled into nasogastric or orogastric tubes in the first 12–24 hours to reduce the incidence of stress ulcers. Other drugs, such as H_2-blockers and proton-pump inhibitors, increase gastric pH and should be avoided; however, if patients are very high risk, a proton-pump inhibitor may be given in conjunction with sucralfate. Metoclopramide is sometimes used to reduce nausea and vomiting when an nasogastric tube is inserted into a patient who is awake.

43. B: Type I atrial flutter (< 350 bpm) can be terminated by rapid atrial pacing. Ventricular tachycardia is treated with rapid ventricular pacing. Usually four pacing wires (positive and negative right atrial and positive and negative right ventricular) are placed during surgery with the atrial wires exiting to the right of the sternum and the ventricular wires exiting to the left. These wires are usually not connected to a pacemaker unless pacing is required, and the ends must be covered and insulated (usually with a sterile needle cap).

44. C: Carpeting poses the risk of static electricity, which can trigger an impulse in epicardial pacing wires. Carpet must be specially treated with a product such as "Static-Guard" if it is used where patients have pacing wires. Other risks include ungrounded electrical equipment and metallic-coated balloons. Dry air during cold weather can also generate static electricity, so air should be humidified. Battery-powered devices, such as shavers, should be used with the patient. Epicardial pacing wires are usually left in place for 24 hours or longer.

45. D: Patients who receive multiple transfusions with citrated blood products must be carefully monitored for hypocalcemia. Calcium is important for transmitting nerve impulses and regulating muscle contraction and relaxation, including the myocardium. Calcium activates enzymes that stimulate chemical reactions and has a role in the coagulation of blood. Values include the following:
- Normal values: 8.2–10.2 mg/dL.
- Hypocalcemia: less than 8.2 mg/dL; critical value: less than 7 mg/dL.
- Hypercalcemia: more than 10.2 mg/dL; critical value: more than 12 mg/dL.
Symptoms include tetany, tingling, seizures, altered mental status, and ventricular tachycardia. Treatment is calcium replacement and vitamin D.

46. B: If a patient fails to respond to atrial pacing or catecholamines (e.g., epinephrine), then ventricular pacing is usually the next step. If the ventricular wires do not function, then transcutaneous pacing may be considered. Sinus bradycardia is a pulse rate of less than 60 bpm. The aim of treatment after cardiopulmonary bypass is to increase the heart rate to about 90 bpm to

maintain adequate cardiac output. Increasing the heart rate improves the contractility of the heart and improves cardiac output.

47. C: Cryoprecipitate is indicated for a patient with significant mediastinal bleeding and a fibrinogen level of less than 100 mg/dL. Platelet transfusion is indicated for bleeding and a platelet count of less than 100,000 µL or suspected platelet dysfunction. Fresh frozen plasma is used to treat an abnormal international normalized ratio. Packed red blood cells are usually administered with bleeding and a hematocrit of less than 26%. Leukocyte-reduced transfusions reduce the risk of infection and have lower mortality rates. Blood filters are commonly used for blood transfusions. Blood warmers should be used for rapid transfusions.

48. B: A β-blocker, such as esmolol, may help to reduce the myocardium's need for oxygen and protect the suture line by lowering the systolic blood pressure. After repair of aortic stenosis, a delayed increase in systolic blood pressure may occur because left ventricular pressure is high. The heart rate should be maintained at 90–100 bpm with adequate preload (pulmonary capillary wedge pressure ≥ 20 mm Hg) with left ventricular hypertrophy, a common condition associated with aortic stenosis.

49. A: When managing hemodynamic problems, an inotropic agent is indicated to treat hypotension, increased pulmonary capillary wedge pressure (PCWP), decreased cardiac output and increased systemic vascular resistance (SVR). If hypertension is present with the other findings the same, a vasodilator is indicated. If all parameters (i.e., blood pressure [BP], PCWP, cardiac output, SVR) are decreased, intravenous fluids are administered. If BP and cardiac output are within normal limits but PCWP and SVR are increased, then a venodilator (nitrate) or diuretic is indicated to stabilize the hemodynamics.

50. A: Patients receiving thoracic epidural analgesia must be monitored carefully for weakness in the lower extremities as an epidural hematoma may develop at the insertion site because of heparinization. Additionally, respiratory depression may occur and delay extubation. Onset of respiratory depression is rapid with fentanyl and sufentanil and delayed with morphine; however, respiratory depression most often occurs with high doses of drugs, such as 4 mg of morphine. Other adverse effects include pruritus, nausea, vomiting, and urinary retention.

Secret Key #1 - Time is Your Greatest Enemy

Pace Yourself

Wear a watch. At the beginning of the test, check the time (or start a chronometer on your watch to count the minutes), and check the time after every few questions to make sure you are "on schedule."

If you are forced to speed up, do it efficiently. Usually one or more answer choices can be eliminated without too much difficulty. Above all, don't panic. Don't speed up and just begin guessing at random choices. By pacing yourself, and continually monitoring your progress against your watch, you will always know exactly how far ahead or behind you are with your available time. If you find that you are one minute behind on the test, don't skip one question without spending any time on it, just to catch back up. Take 15 fewer seconds on the next four questions, and after four questions you'll have caught back up. Once you catch back up, you can continue working each problem at your normal pace.

Furthermore, don't dwell on the problems that you were rushed on. If a problem was taking up too much time and you made a hurried guess, it must be difficult. The difficult questions are the ones you are most likely to miss anyway, so it isn't a big loss. It is better to end with more time than you need than to run out of time.

Lastly, sometimes it is beneficial to slow down if you are constantly getting ahead of time. You are always more likely to catch a careless mistake by working more slowly than quickly, and among very high-scoring test takers (those who are likely to have lots of time left over), careless errors affect the score more than mastery of material.

Secret Key #2 - Guessing is not Guesswork

You probably know that guessing is a good idea. Unlike other standardized tests, there is no penalty for getting a wrong answer. Even if you have no idea about a question, you still have a 20-25% chance of getting it right.

Most test takers do not understand the impact that proper guessing can have on their score. Unless you score extremely high, guessing will significantly contribute to your final score.

Monkeys Take the Test

What most test takers don't realize is that to insure that 20-25% chance, you have to guess randomly. If you put 20 monkeys in a room to take this test, assuming they answered once per question and behaved themselves, on average they would get 20-25% of the questions correct. Put 20 test takers in the room, and the average will be much lower among guessed questions. Why?
  1. The test writers intentionally write deceptive answer choices that "look" right. A test taker has no idea about a question, so he picks the "best looking" answer, which is often wrong. The monkey has no idea what looks good and what doesn't, so it will consistently be right about 20-25% of the time.

2. Test takers will eliminate answer choices from the guessing pool based on a hunch or intuition. Simple but correct answers often get excluded, leaving a 0% chance of being correct. The monkey has no clue, and often gets lucky with the best choice.

This is why the process of elimination endorsed by most test courses is flawed and detrimental to your performance. Test takers don't guess; they make an ignorant stab in the dark that is usually worse than random.

$5 Challenge

Let me introduce one of the most valuable ideas of this course—the $5 challenge:

You only mark your "best guess" if you are willing to bet $5 on it.
You only eliminate choices from guessing if you are willing to bet $5 on it.

Why $5? Five dollars is an amount of money that is small yet not insignificant, and can really add up fast (20 questions could cost you $100). Likewise, each answer choice on one question of the test will have a small impact on your overall score, but it can really add up to a lot of points in the end.

The process of elimination IS valuable. The following shows your chance of guessing it right:

If you eliminate wrong answer choices until only this many remain:	Chance of getting it correct:
1	100%
2	50%
3	33%

However, if you accidentally eliminate the right answer or go on a hunch for an incorrect answer, your chances drop dramatically—to 0%. By guessing among all the answer choices, you are GUARANTEED to have a shot at the right answer.

That's why the $5 test is so valuable. If you give up the advantage and safety of a pure guess, it had better be worth the risk.

What we still haven't covered is how to be sure that whatever guess you make is truly random. Here's the easiest way:

Always pick the first answer choice among those remaining.

Such a technique means that you have decided, **before you see a single test question**, exactly how you are going to guess, and since the order of choices tells you nothing about which one is correct, this guessing technique is perfectly random.

This section is not meant to scare you away from making educated guesses or eliminating choices; you just need to define when a choice is worth eliminating. The $5 test, along with a pre-defined random guessing strategy, is the best way to make sure you reap all of the benefits of guessing.

Secret Key #3 - Practice Smarter, Not Harder

Many test takers delay the test preparation process because they dread the awful amounts of practice time they think necessary to succeed on the test. We have refined an effective method that will take you only a fraction of the time.

There are a number of "obstacles" in the path to success. Among these are answering questions, finishing in time, and mastering test-taking strategies. All must be executed on the day of the test at peak performance, or your score will suffer. The test is a mental marathon that has a large impact on your future.

Just like a marathon runner, it is important to work your way up to the full challenge. So first you just worry about questions, and then time, and finally strategy:

Success Strategy

1. Find a good source for practice tests.
2. If you are willing to make a larger time investment, consider using more than one study guide. Often the different approaches of multiple authors will help you "get" difficult concepts.
3. Take a practice test with no time constraints, with all study helps, "open book." Take your time with questions and focus on applying strategies.
4. Take a practice test with time constraints, with all guides, "open book."
5. Take a final practice test without open material and with time limits.

If you have time to take more practice tests, just repeat step 5. By gradually exposing yourself to the full rigors of the test environment, you will condition your mind to the stress of test day and maximize your success.

Secret Key #4 - **Prepare, Don't Procrastinate**

Let me state an obvious fact: if you take the test three times, you will probably get three different scores. This is due to the way you feel on test day, the level of preparedness you have, and the version of the test you see. Despite the test writers' claims to the contrary, some versions of the test WILL be easier for you than others.

Since your future depends so much on your score, you should maximize your chances of success. In order to maximize the likelihood of success, you've got to prepare in advance. This means taking practice tests and spending time learning the information and test taking strategies you will need to succeed.

Never go take the actual test as a "practice" test, expecting that you can just take it again if you need to. Take all the practice tests you can on your own, but when you go to take the official test, be prepared, be focused, and do your best the first time!

Secret Key #5 - Test Yourself

Everyone knows that time is money. There is no need to spend too much of your time or too little of your time preparing for the test. You should only spend as much of your precious time preparing as is necessary for you to get the score you need.

Once you have taken a practice test under real conditions of time constraints, then you will know if you are ready for the test or not.

If you have scored extremely high the first time that you take the practice test, then there is not much point in spending countless hours studying. You are already there.

Benchmark your abilities by retaking practice tests and seeing how much you have improved. Once you consistently score high enough to guarantee success, then you are ready.

If you have scored well below where you need, then knuckle down and begin studying in earnest. Check your improvement regularly through the use of practice tests under real conditions. Above all, don't worry, panic, or give up. The key is perseverance!

Then, when you go to take the test, remain confident and remember how well you did on the practice tests. If you can score high enough on a practice test, then you can do the same on the real thing.

General Strategies

The most important thing you can do is to ignore your fears and jump into the test immediately. Do not be overwhelmed by any strange-sounding terms. You have to jump into the test like jumping into a pool—all at once is the easiest way.

Make Predictions

As you read and understand the question, try to guess what the answer will be. Remember that several of the answer choices are wrong, and once you begin reading them, your mind will immediately become cluttered with answer choices designed to throw you off. Your mind is typically the most focused immediately after you have read the question and digested its contents. If you can, try to predict what the correct answer will be. You may be surprised at what you can predict.

Quickly scan the choices and see if your prediction is in the listed answer choices. If it is, then you can be quite confident that you have the right answer. It still won't hurt to check the other answer choices, but most of the time, you've got it!

Answer the Question

It may seem obvious to only pick answer choices that answer the question, but the test writers can create some excellent answer choices that are wrong. Don't pick an answer just because it sounds right, or you believe it to be true. It MUST answer the question. Once you've made your selection, always go back and check it against the question and make sure that you didn't misread the question and that the answer choice does answer the question posed.

Benchmark

After you read the first answer choice, decide if you think it sounds correct or not. If it doesn't, move on to the next answer choice. If it does, mentally mark that answer choice. This doesn't mean that you've definitely selected it as your answer choice, it just means that it's the best you've seen thus far. Go ahead and read the next choice. If the next choice is worse than the one you've already selected, keep going to the next answer choice. If the next choice is better than the choice you've already selected, mentally mark the new answer choice as your best guess.

The first answer choice that you select becomes your standard. Every other answer choice must be benchmarked against that standard. That choice is correct until proven otherwise by another answer choice beating it out. Once you've decided that no other answer choice seems as good, do one final check to ensure that your answer choice answers the question posed.

Valid Information

Don't discount any of the information provided in the question. Every piece of information may be necessary to determine the correct answer. None of the information in the question is there to throw you off (while the answer choices will certainly have information to throw you off). If two seemingly unrelated topics are discussed, don't ignore either. You can be confident there is a relationship, or it wouldn't be included in the question, and you are probably going to have to determine what is that relationship to find the answer.

Avoid "Fact Traps"

Don't get distracted by a choice that is factually true. Your search is for the answer that answers the question. Stay focused and don't fall for an answer that is true but irrelevant. Always go back to the question and make sure you're choosing an answer that actually answers the question and is not just a true statement. An answer can be factually correct, but it MUST answer the question asked. Additionally, two answers can both be seemingly correct, so be sure to read all of the answer choices, and make sure that you get the one that BEST answers the question.

Milk the Question

Some of the questions may throw you completely off. They might deal with a subject you have not been exposed to, or one that you haven't reviewed in years. While your lack of knowledge about the subject will be a hindrance, the question itself can give you many clues that will help you find the correct answer. Read the question carefully and look for clues. Watch particularly for adjectives and nouns describing difficult terms or words that you don't recognize. Regardless of whether you completely understand a word or not, replacing it with a synonym, either provided or one you more familiar with, may help you to understand what the questions are asking. Rather than wracking your mind about specific detailed information concerning a difficult term or word, try to use mental substitutes that are easier to understand.

The Trap of Familiarity

Don't just choose a word because you recognize it. On difficult questions, you may not recognize a number of words in the answer choices. The test writers don't put "make-believe" words on the test, so don't think that just because you only recognize all the words in one answer choice that that answer choice must be correct. If you only recognize words in one answer choice, then focus on that one. Is it correct? Try your best to determine if it is correct. If it is, that's great. If not, eliminate it. Each word and answer choice you eliminate increases your chances of getting the question correct, even if you then have to guess among the unfamiliar choices.

Eliminate Answers

Eliminate choices as soon as you realize they are wrong. But be careful! Make sure you consider all of the possible answer choices. Just because one appears right, doesn't mean that the next one won't be even better! The test writers will usually put more than one good answer choice for every question, so read all of them. Don't worry if you are stuck between two that seem right. By getting down to just two remaining possible choices, your odds are now 50/50. Rather than wasting too much time, play the odds. You are guessing, but guessing wisely because you've been able to knock out some of the answer choices that you know are wrong. If you are eliminating choices and realize that the last answer choice you are left with is also obviously wrong, don't panic. Start over and consider each choice again. There may easily be something that you missed the first time and will realize on the second pass.

Tough Questions

If you are stumped on a problem or it appears too hard or too difficult, don't waste time. Move on! Remember though, if you can quickly check for obviously incorrect answer choices, your chances of guessing correctly are greatly improved. Before you completely give up, at least try to knock out a couple of possible answers. Eliminate what you can and then guess at the remaining answer choices before moving on.

Brainstorm

If you get stuck on a difficult question, spend a few seconds quickly brainstorming. Run through the complete list of possible answer choices. Look at each choice and ask yourself, "Could this answer the question satisfactorily?" Go through each answer choice and consider it independently of the others. By systematically going through all possibilities, you may find something that you would otherwise overlook. Remember though that when you get stuck, it's important to try to keep moving.

Read Carefully

Understand the problem. Read the question and answer choices carefully. Don't miss the question because you misread the terms. You have plenty of time to read each question thoroughly and make sure you understand what is being asked. Yet a happy medium must be attained, so don't waste too much time. You must read carefully, but efficiently.

Face Value

When in doubt, use common sense. Always accept the situation in the problem at face value. Don't read too much into it. These problems will not require you to make huge leaps of logic. The test writers aren't trying to throw you off with a cheap trick. If you have to go beyond creativity and make a leap of logic in order to have an answer choice answer the question, then you should look at the other answer choices. Don't overcomplicate the problem by creating theoretical relationships or explanations that will warp time or space. These are normal problems rooted in reality. It's just that the applicable relationship or explanation may not be readily apparent and you have to figure things out. Use your common sense to interpret anything that isn't clear.

Prefixes

If you're having trouble with a word in the question or answer choices, try dissecting it. Take advantage of every clue that the word might include. Prefixes and suffixes can be a huge help. Usually they allow you to determine a basic meaning. Pre- means before, post- means after, pro - is positive, de- is negative. From these prefixes and suffixes, you can get an idea of the general meaning of the word and try to put it into context. Beware though of any traps. Just because con- is the opposite of pro-, doesn't necessarily mean congress is the opposite of progress!

Hedge Phrases

Watch out for critical hedge phrases, led off with words such as "likely," "may," "can," "sometimes," "often," "almost," "mostly," "usually," "generally," "rarely," and "sometimes." Question writers insert these hedge phrases to cover every possibility. Often an answer choice will be wrong simply because it leaves no room for exception. Unless the situation calls for them, avoid answer choices that have definitive words like "exactly," and "always."

Switchback Words

Stay alert for "switchbacks." These are the words and phrases frequently used to alert you to shifts in thought. The most common switchback word is "but." Others include "although," "however," "nevertheless," "on the other hand," "even though," "while," "in spite of," "despite," and "regardless of."

New Information

Correct answer choices will rarely have completely new information included. Answer choices typically are straightforward reflections of the material asked about and will directly relate to the question. If a new piece of information is included in an answer choice that doesn't even seem to relate to the topic being asked about, then that answer choice is likely incorrect. All of the information needed to answer the question is usually provided for you in the question. You should not have to make guesses that are unsupported or choose answer choices that require unknown information that cannot be reasoned from what is given.

Time Management

On technical questions, don't get lost on the technical terms. Don't spend too much time on any one question. If you don't know what a term means, then odds are you aren't going to get much further since you don't have a dictionary. You should be able to immediately recognize whether or not you know a term. If you don't, work with the other clues that you have—the other answer choices and terms provided—but don't waste too much time trying to figure out a difficult term that you don't know.

Contextual Clues

Look for contextual clues. An answer can be right but not the correct answer. The contextual clues will help you find the answer that is most right and is correct. Understand the context in which a phrase or statement is made. This will help you make important distinctions.

Don't Panic

Panicking will not answer any questions for you; therefore, it isn't helpful. When you first see the question, if your mind goes blank, take a deep breath. Force yourself to mechanically go through the steps of solving the problem using the strategies you've learned.

Pace Yourself

Don't get clock fever. It's easy to be overwhelmed when you're looking at a page full of questions, your mind is full of random thoughts and feeling confused, and the clock is ticking down faster than you would like. Calm down and maintain the pace that you have set for yourself. As long as you are on track by monitoring your pace, you are guaranteed to have enough time for yourself. When you get to the last few minutes of the test, it may seem like you won't have enough time left, but if you only have as many questions as you should have left at that point, then you're right on track!

Answer Selection

The best way to pick an answer choice is to eliminate all of those that are wrong, until only one is left and confirm that is the correct answer. Sometimes though, an answer choice may immediately look right. Be careful! Take a second to make sure that the other choices are not equally obvious. Don't make a hasty mistake. There are only two times that you should stop before checking other answers. First is when you are positive that the answer choice you have selected is correct. Second is when time is almost out and you have to make a quick guess!

Check Your Work

Since you will probably not know every term listed and the answer to every question, it is important that you get credit for the ones that you do know. Don't miss any questions through careless mistakes. If at all possible, try to take a second to look back over your answer selection and make sure you've selected the correct answer choice and haven't made a costly careless mistake (such as marking an answer choice that you didn't mean to mark). The time it takes for this quick double check should more than pay for itself in caught mistakes.

Beware of Directly Quoted Answers

Sometimes an answer choice will repeat word for word a portion of the question or reference section. However, beware of such exact duplication. It may be a trap! More than likely, the correct choice will paraphrase or summarize a point, rather than being exactly the same wording.

Slang

Scientific sounding answers are better than slang ones. An answer choice that begins "To compare the outcomes…" is much more likely to be correct than one that begins "Because some people insisted…"

Extreme Statements

Avoid wild answers that throw out highly controversial ideas that are proclaimed as established fact. An answer choice that states the "process should be used in certain situations, if…" is much more likely to be correct than one that states the "process should be discontinued completely." The first is a calm rational statement and doesn't even make a definitive, uncompromising stance, using a hedge word "if" to provide wiggle room, whereas the second choice is a radical idea and far more extreme.

Answer Choice Families

When you have two or more answer choices that are direct opposites or parallels, one of them is usually the correct answer. For instance, if one answer choice states "x increases" and another answer choice states "x decreases" or "y increases," then those two or three answer choices are very similar in construction and fall into the same family of answer choices. A family of answer choices consists of two or three answer choices, very similar in construction, but often with directly opposite meanings. Usually the correct answer choice will be in that family of answer choices. The "odd man out" or answer choice that doesn't seem to fit the parallel construction of the other answer choices is more likely to be incorrect.

Special Report: What Your Test Score Will Tell You About Your IQ

Did you know that most standardized tests correlate very strongly with IQ? In fact, your general intelligence is a better predictor of your success than any other factor, and most tests intentionally measure this trait to some degree to ensure that those selected by the test are truly qualified for the test's purposes.

Before we can delve into the relation between your test score and IQ, I will first have to explain what exactly is IQ. Here's the formula:

Your IQ = 100 + (Number of standard deviations below or above the average)*15

Now, let's define standard deviations by using an example. If we have 5 people with 5 different heights, then first we calculate the average. Let's say the average was 65 inches. The standard deviation is the "average distance" away from the average of each of the members. It is a direct measure of variability. If the 5 people included Jackie Chan and Shaquille O'Neal, obviously there's a lot more variability in that group than a group of 5 sisters who are all within 6 inches in height of each other. The standard deviation uses a number to characterize the average range of difference within a group.

A convenient feature of most groups is that they have a "normal" distribution. It makes sense that most things would be normal, right? Without getting into a bunch of statistical mumbo-jumbo, you just need to know that if you know the average of the group and the standard deviation, you can successfully predict someone's percentile rank in the group.

Confused? Let me give you an example. If instead of 5 people's heights, we had 100 people, we could figure out their rank in height JUST by knowing the average, standard deviation, and their height. We wouldn't need to know each person's height and manually rank them, we could just predict their rank based on three numbers.

What this means is that you can take your PERCENTILE rank that is often given with your test and relate this to your RELATIVE IQ of people taking the test - that is, your IQ relative to the people taking the test. Obviously, there's no way to know your actual IQ because the people taking a standardized test are usually not very good samples of the general population. Many of those with extremely low IQ's never achieve a level of success or competency necessary to complete a typical standardized test. In fact, professional psychologists who measure IQ actually have to use non-written tests that can fairly measure the IQ of those not able to complete a traditional test.

The bottom line is to not take your test score too seriously, but it is fun to compute your "relative IQ" among the people who took the test with you. I've done the calculations below. Just look up your percentile rank in the left and then you'll see your "relative IQ" for your test in the right hand column.

Percentile Rank	Your Relative IQ		Percentile Rank	Your Relative IQ
99	135		59	103
98	131		58	103
97	128		57	103
96	126		56	102
95	125		55	102
94	123		54	102
93	122		53	101
92	121		52	101
91	120		51	100
90	119		50	100
89	118		49	100
88	118		48	99
87	117		47	99
86	116		46	98
85	116		45	98
84	115		44	98
83	114		43	97
82	114		42	97
81	113		41	97
80	113		40	96
79	112		39	96
78	112		38	95
77	111		37	95
76	111		36	95
75	110		35	94
74	110		34	94
73	109		33	93
72	109		32	93
71	108		31	93
70	108		30	92
69	107		29	92
68	107		28	91
67	107		27	91
66	106		26	90
65	106		25	90
64	105		24	89
63	105		23	89
62	105		22	88
61	104		21	88
60	104		20	87

Special Report: What is Test Anxiety and How to Overcome It?

The very nature of tests caters to some level of anxiety, nervousness, or tension, just as we feel for any important event that occurs in our lives. A little bit of anxiety or nervousness can be a good thing. It helps us with motivation, and makes achievement just that much sweeter. However, too much anxiety can be a problem, especially if it hinders our ability to function and perform.

"Test anxiety," is the term that refers to the emotional reactions that some test-takers experience when faced with a test or exam. Having a fear of testing and exams is based upon a rational fear, since the test-taker's performance can shape the course of an academic career. Nevertheless, experiencing excessive fear of examinations will only interfere with the test-taker's ability to perform and chance to be successful.

There are a large variety of causes that can contribute to the development and sensation of test anxiety. These include, but are not limited to, lack of preparation and worrying about issues surrounding the test.

Lack of Preparation

Lack of preparation can be identified by the following behaviors or situations:

Not scheduling enough time to study, and therefore cramming the night before the test or exam
Managing time poorly, to create the sensation that there is not enough time to do everything
Failing to organize the text information in advance, so that the study material consists of the entire text and not simply the pertinent information
Poor overall studying habits

Worrying, on the other hand, can be related to both the test taker, or many other factors around him/her that will be affected by the results of the test. These include worrying about:

Previous performances on similar exams, or exams in general
How friends and other students are achieving
The negative consequences that will result from a poor grade or failure

There are three primary elements to test anxiety. Physical components, which involve the same typical bodily reactions as those to acute anxiety (to be discussed below). Emotional factors have to do with fear or panic. Mental or cognitive issues concerning attention spans and memory abilities.

Physical Signals

There are many different symptoms of test anxiety, and these are not limited to mental and emotional strain. Frequently there are a range of physical signals that will let a test taker know that he/she is suffering from test anxiety. These bodily changes can include the following:

Perspiring
Sweaty palms
Wet, trembling hands
Nausea
Dry mouth
A knot in the stomach
Headache
Faintness
Muscle tension
Aching shoulders, back and neck
Rapid heart beat
Feeling too hot/cold

To recognize the sensation of test anxiety, a test-taker should monitor him/herself for the following sensations:

The physical distress symptoms as listed above
Emotional sensitivity, expressing emotional feelings such as the need to cry or laugh too much, or a sensation of anger or helplessness
A decreased ability to think, causing the test-taker to blank out or have racing thoughts that are hard to organize or control.

Though most students will feel some level of anxiety when faced with a test or exam, the majority can cope with that anxiety and maintain it at a manageable level. However, those who cannot are faced with a very real and very serious condition, which can and should be controlled for the immeasurable benefit of this sufferer.

Naturally, these sensations lead to negative results for the testing experience. The most common effects of test anxiety have to do with nervousness and mental blocking.

Nervousness

Nervousness can appear in several different levels:

The test-taker's difficulty, or even inability to read and understand the questions on the test
The difficulty or inability to organize thoughts to a coherent form
The difficulty or inability to recall key words and concepts relating to the testing questions (especially essays)
The receipt of poor grades on a test, though the test material was well known by the test taker

Conversely, a person may also experience mental blocking, which involves:

Blanking out on test questions
Only remembering the correct answers to the questions when the test has already finished.

Fortunately for test anxiety sufferers, beating these feelings, to a large degree, has to do with proper preparation. When a test taker has a feeling of preparedness, then anxiety will be dramatically lessened.

The first step to resolving anxiety issues is to distinguish which of the two types of anxiety are being suffered. If the anxiety is a direct result of a lack of preparation, this should be considered a normal reaction, and the anxiety level (as opposed to the test results) shouldn't be anything to worry about. However, if, when adequately prepared, the test-taker still panics, blanks out, or seems to overreact, this is not a fully rational reaction. While this can be considered normal too, there are many ways to combat and overcome these effects.

Remember that anxiety cannot be entirely eliminated, however, there are ways to minimize it, to make the anxiety easier to manage. Preparation is one of the best ways to minimize test anxiety. Therefore the following techniques are wise in order to best fight off any anxiety that may want to build.

To begin with, try to avoid cramming before a test, whenever it is possible. By trying to memorize an entire term's worth of information in one day, you'll be shocking your system, and not giving yourself a very good chance to absorb the information. This is an easy path to anxiety, so for those who suffer from test anxiety, cramming should not even be considered an option.

Instead of cramming, work throughout the semester to combine all of the material which is presented throughout the semester, and work on it gradually as the course goes by, making sure to master the main concepts first, leaving minor details for a week or so before the test.

To study for the upcoming exam, be sure to pose questions that may be on the examination, to gauge the ability to answer them by integrating the ideas from your texts, notes and lectures, as well as any supplementary readings.

If it is truly impossible to cover all of the information that was covered in that particular term, concentrate on the most important portions that can be covered very well. Learn these concepts as best as possible, so that when the test comes, a goal can be made to use these concepts as presentations of your knowledge.

In addition to study habits, changes in attitude are critical to beating a struggle with test anxiety. In fact, an improvement of the perspective over the entire test-taking experience can actually help a test taker to enjoy studying and therefore improve the overall experience. Be certain not to overemphasize the significance of the grade - know that the result of the test is neither a reflection of self worth, nor is it a measure of intelligence; one grade will not predict a person's future success.

To improve an overall testing outlook, the following steps should be tried:

Keeping in mind that the most reasonable expectation for taking a test is to expect to try to demonstrate as much of what you know as you possibly can.

Reminding ourselves that a test is only one test; this is not the only one, and there will be others.

The thought of thinking of oneself in an irrational, all-or-nothing term should be avoided at all costs.

A reward should be designated for after the test, so there's something to look forward to. Whether it be going to a movie, going out to eat, or simply visiting friends, schedule it in advance, and do it no matter what result is expected on the exam.

Test-takers should also keep in mind that the basics are some of the most important things, even beyond anti-anxiety techniques and studying. Never neglect the basic social, emotional and biological needs, in order to try to absorb information. In order to best achieve, these three factors must be held as just as important as the studying itself.

Study Steps

Remember the following important steps for studying:

Maintain healthy nutrition and exercise habits. Continue both your recreational activities and social pass times. These both contribute to your physical and emotional well being.
Be certain to get a good amount of sleep, especially the night before the test, because when you're overtired you are not able to perform to the best of your best ability.
Keep the studying pace to a moderate level by taking breaks when they are needed, and varying the work whenever possible, to keep the mind fresh instead of getting bored.
When enough studying has been done that all the material that can be learned has been learned, and the test taker is prepared for the test, stop studying and do something relaxing such as listening to music, watching a movie, or taking a warm bubble bath.

There are also many other techniques to minimize the uneasiness or apprehension that is experienced along with test anxiety before, during, or even after the examination. In fact, there are a great deal of things that can be done to stop anxiety from interfering with lifestyle and performance. Again, remember that anxiety will not be eliminated entirely, and it shouldn't be. Otherwise that "up" feeling for exams would not exist, and most of us depend on that sensation to perform better than usual. However, this anxiety has to be at a level that is manageable.

Of course, as we have just discussed, being prepared for the exam is half the battle right away. Attending all classes, finding out what knowledge will be expected on the exam, and knowing the exam schedules are easy steps to lowering anxiety. Keeping up with work will remove the need to cram, and efficient study habits will eliminate wasted time. Studying should be done in an ideal location for concentration, so that it is simple to become interested in the material and give it complete attention. A method such as SQ3R (Survey, Question, Read, Recite, Review) is a wonderful key to follow to make sure that the study habits are as effective as possible, especially in the case of learning from a textbook. Flashcards are great techniques for memorization. Learning to take good notes will mean that notes will be full of useful information, so that less sifting will need to be done to seek out what is pertinent for studying. Reviewing notes after class and then again on occasion will keep the information fresh in the mind. From notes that have been taken summary sheets and outlines can be made for simpler reviewing.

A study group can also be a very motivational and helpful place to study, as there will be a sharing of ideas, all of the minds can work together, to make sure that everyone understands, and the studying will be made more interesting because it will be a social occasion.

Basically, though, as long as the test-taker remains organized and self confident, with efficient study habits, less time will need to be spent studying, and higher grades will be achieved.

To become self confident, there are many useful steps. The first of these is "self talk." It has been shown through extensive research, that self-talk for students who suffer from test anxiety, should be well monitored, in order to make sure that it contributes to self confidence as opposed to sinking the student. Frequently the self talk of test-anxious students is negative or self-defeating, thinking that everyone else is smarter and faster, that they always mess up, and that if they don't do well, they'll fail the entire course. It is important to decreasing anxiety that awareness is made of self talk. Try writing any negative self thoughts and then disputing them with a positive statement instead. Begin self-encouragement as though it was a friend speaking. Repeat positive statements to help reprogram the mind to believing in successes instead of failures.

Helpful Techniques

Other extremely helpful techniques include:

Self-visualization of doing well and reaching goals
While aiming for an "A" level of understanding, don't try to "overprotect" by setting your expectations lower. This will only convince the mind to stop studying in order to meet the lower expectations.
Don't make comparisons with the results or habits of other students. These are individual factors, and different things work for different people, causing different results.
Strive to become an expert in learning what works well, and what can be done in order to improve. Consider collecting this data in a journal.
Create rewards for after studying instead of doing things before studying that will only turn into avoidance behaviors.
Make a practice of relaxing - by using methods such as progressive relaxation, self-hypnosis, guided imagery, etc - in order to make relaxation an automatic sensation.
Work on creating a state of relaxed concentration so that concentrating will take on the focus of the mind, so that none will be wasted on worrying.
Take good care of the physical self by eating well and getting enough sleep.
Plan in time for exercise and stick to this plan.

Beyond these techniques, there are other methods to be used before, during and after the test that will help the test-taker perform well in addition to overcoming anxiety.

Before the exam comes the academic preparation. This involves establishing a study schedule and beginning at least one week before the actual date of the test. By doing this, the anxiety of not having enough time to study for the test will be automatically eliminated. Moreover, this will make the studying a much more effective experience, ensuring that the learning will be an easier process. This relieves much undue pressure on the test-taker.

Summary sheets, note cards, and flash cards with the main concepts and examples of these main concepts should be prepared in advance of the actual studying time. A topic should never be eliminated from this process. By omitting a topic because it isn't expected to be on the test is only setting up the test-taker for anxiety should it actually appear on the exam. Utilize the course syllabus for laying out the topics that should be studied. Carefully go over the notes that were made in class, paying special attention to any of the issues that the professor took special care to emphasize while lecturing in class. In the textbooks, use the chapter review, or if possible, the chapter tests, to begin your review.

It may even be possible to ask the instructor what information will be covered on the exam, or what the format of the exam will be (for example, multiple choice, essay, free form, true-false). Additionally, see if it is possible to find out how many questions will be on the test. If a review sheet or sample test has been offered by the professor, make good use of it, above anything else, for the preparation for the test. Another great resource for getting to know the examination is reviewing tests from previous semesters. Use these tests to review, and aim to achieve a 100% score on each of the possible topics. With a few exceptions, the goal that you set for yourself is the highest one that you will reach.

Take all of the questions that were assigned as homework, and rework them to any other possible course material. The more problems reworked, the more skill and confidence will form as a result. When forming the solution to a problem, write out each of the steps. Don't simply do head work. By doing as many steps on paper as possible, much clarification and therefore confidence will be formed. Do this with as many homework problems as possible, before checking the answers. By checking the answer after each problem, a reinforcement will exist, that will not be on the exam. Study situations should be as exam-like as possible, to prime the test-taker's system for the experience. By waiting to check the answers at the end, a psychological advantage will be formed, to decrease the stress factor.

Another fantastic reason for not cramming is the avoidance of confusion in concepts, especially when it comes to mathematics. 8-10 hours of study will become one hundred percent more effective if it is spread out over a week or at least several days, instead of doing it all in one sitting. Recognize that the human brain requires time in order to assimilate new material, so frequent breaks and a span of study time over several days will be much more beneficial.

Additionally, don't study right up until the point of the exam. Studying should stop a minimum of one hour before the exam begins. This allows the brain to rest and put things in their proper order. This will also provide the time to become as relaxed as possible when going into the examination room. The test-taker will also have time to eat well and eat sensibly. Know that the brain needs food as much as the rest of the body. With enough food and enough sleep, as well as a relaxed attitude, the body and the mind are primed for success.

Avoid any anxious classmates who are talking about the exam. These students only spread anxiety, and are not worth sharing the anxious sentimentalities.

Before the test also involves creating a positive attitude, so mental preparation should also be a point of concentration. There are many keys to creating a positive attitude. Should fears become rushing in, make a visualization of taking the exam, doing well, and seeing an A written on the paper. Write out a list of affirmations that will bring a feeling of confidence, such as "I am doing well in my English class," "I studied well and know my material," "I enjoy this class." Even if the affirmations aren't believed at first, it sends a positive message to the subconscious which will result in an alteration of the overall belief system, which is the system that creates reality.

If a sensation of panic begins, work with the fear and imagine the very worst! Work through the entire scenario of not passing the test, failing the entire course, and dropping out of school, followed by not getting a job, and pushing a shopping cart through the dark alley where you'll live. This will place things into perspective! Then, practice deep breathing and create a visualization of the opposite situation - achieving an "A" on the exam, passing the entire course, receiving the degree at a graduation ceremony.

On the day of the test, there are many things to be done to ensure the best results, as well as the most calm outlook. The following stages are suggested in order to maximize test-taking potential:

Begin the examination day with a moderate breakfast, and avoid any coffee or beverages with caffeine if the test taker is prone to jitters. Even people who are used to managing caffeine can feel jittery or light-headed when it is taken on a test day.
Attempt to do something that is relaxing before the examination begins. As last minute cramming clouds the mastering of overall concepts, it is better to use this time to create a calming outlook.
Be certain to arrive at the test location well in advance, in order to provide time to select a location that is away from doors, windows and other distractions, as well as giving enough time to relax before the test begins.
Keep away from anxiety generating classmates who will upset the sensation of stability and relaxation that is being attempted before the exam.
Should the waiting period before the exam begins cause anxiety, create a self-distraction by reading a light magazine or something else that is relaxing and simple.

During the exam itself, read the entire exam from beginning to end, and find out how much time should be allotted to each individual problem. Once writing the exam, should more time be taken for a problem, it should be abandoned, in order to begin another problem. If there is time at the end, the unfinished problem can always be returned to and completed.

Read the instructions very carefully - twice - so that unpleasant surprises won't follow during or after the exam has ended.

When writing the exam, pretend that the situation is actually simply the completion of homework within a library, or at home. This will assist in forming a relaxed atmosphere, and will allow the brain extra focus for the complex thinking function.

Begin the exam with all of the questions with which the most confidence is felt. This will build the confidence level regarding the entire exam and will begin a quality momentum. This will also create encouragement for trying the problems where uncertainty resides.

Going with the "gut instinct" is always the way to go when solving a problem. Second guessing should be avoided at all costs. Have confidence in the ability to do well.

For essay questions, create an outline in advance that will keep the mind organized and make certain that all of the points are remembered. For multiple choice, read every answer, even if the correct one has been spotted - a better one may exist.

Continue at a pace that is reasonable and not rushed, in order to be able to work carefully. Provide enough time to go over the answers at the end, to check for small errors that can be corrected.

Should a feeling of panic begin, breathe deeply, and think of the feeling of the body releasing sand through its pores. Visualize a calm, peaceful place, and include all of the sights, sounds and sensations of this image. Continue the deep breathing, and take a few minutes to continue this with closed eyes. When all is well again, return to the test.

If a "blanking" occurs for a certain question, skip it and move on to the next question. There will be time to return to the other question later. Get everything done that can be done, first, to guarantee all the grades that can be compiled, and to build all of the confidence possible. Then return to the weaker questions to build the marks from there.

Remember, one's own reality can be created, so as long as the belief is there, success will follow. And remember: anxiety can happen later, right now, there's an exam to be written!

After the examination is complete, whether there is a feeling for a good grade or a bad grade, don't dwell on the exam, and be certain to follow through on the reward that was promised...and enjoy it! Don't dwell on any mistakes that have been made, as there is nothing that can be done at this point anyway.

Additionally, don't begin to study for the next test right away. Do something relaxing for a while, and let the mind relax and prepare itself to begin absorbing information again.

From the results of the exam - both the grade and the entire experience, be certain to learn from what has gone on. Perfect studying habits and work some more on confidence in order to make the next examination experience even better than the last one.

Learn to avoid places where openings occurred for laziness, procrastination and day dreaming.

Use the time between this exam and the next one to better learn to relax, even learning to relax on cue, so that any anxiety can be controlled during the next exam. Learn how to relax the body. Slouch in your chair if that helps. Tighten and then relax all of the different muscle groups, one group at a time, beginning with the feet and then working all the way up to the neck and face. This will ultimately relax the muscles more than they were to begin with. Learn how to breathe deeply and comfortably, and focus on this breathing going in and out as a relaxing thought. With every exhale, repeat the word "relax."

As common as test anxiety is, it is very possible to overcome it. Make yourself one of the test-takers who overcome this frustrating hindrance.

Special Report: Retaking the Test: What Are Your Chances at Improving Your Score?

After going through the experience of taking a major test, many test takers feel that once is enough. The test usually comes during a period of transition in the test taker's life, and taking the test is only one of a series of important events. With so many distractions and conflicting recommendations, it may be difficult for a test taker to rationally determine whether or not he should retake the test after viewing his scores.

The importance of the test usually only adds to the burden of the retake decision. However, don't be swayed by emotion. There a few simple questions that you can ask yourself to guide you as you try to determine whether a retake would improve your score:

1. What went wrong? Why wasn't your score what you expected?

Can you point to a single factor or problem that you feel caused the low score? Were you sick on test day? Was there an emotional upheaval in your life that caused a distraction? Were you late for the test or not able to use the full time allotment? If you can point to any of these specific, individual problems, then a retake should definitely be considered.

2. Is there enough time to improve?

Many problems that may show up in your score report may take a lot of time for improvement. A deficiency in a particular math skill may require weeks or months of tutoring and studying to improve. If you have enough time to improve an identified weakness, then a retake should definitely be considered.

3. How will additional scores be used? Will a score average, highest score, or most recent score be used?

Different test scores may be handled completely differently. If you've taken the test multiple times, sometimes your highest score is used, sometimes your average score is computed and used, and sometimes your most recent score is used. Make sure you understand what method will be used to evaluate your scores, and use that to help you determine whether a retake should be considered.

4. Are my practice test scores significantly higher than my actual test score?

If you have taken a lot of practice tests and are consistently scoring at a much higher level than your actual test score, then you should consider a retake. However, if you've taken five practice tests and only one of your scores was higher than your actual test score, or if your practice test scores were only slightly higher than your actual test score, then it is unlikely that you will significantly increase your score.

5. Do I need perfect scores or will I be able to live with this score? Will this score still allow me to follow my dreams?

What kind of score is acceptable to you? Is your current score "good enough?" Do you have to have a certain score in order to pursue the future of your dreams? If you won't be happy with your current score, and there's no way that you could live with it, then you should consider a retake. However, don't get your hopes up. If you are looking for significant improvement, that may or may not be possible. But if you won't be happy otherwise, it is at least worth the effort. Remember that there are other considerations. To achieve your dream, it is likely that your grades may also be taken into account. A great test score is usually not the only thing necessary to succeed. Make sure that you aren't overemphasizing the importance of a high test score.

Furthermore, a retake does not always result in a higher score. Some test takers will score lower on a retake, rather than higher. One study shows that one-fourth of test takers will achieve a significant improvement in test score, while one-sixth of test takers will actually show a decrease. While this shows that most test takers will improve, the majority will only improve their scores a little and a retake may not be worth the test taker's effort.

Finally, if a test is taken only once and is considered in the added context of good grades on the part of a test taker, the person reviewing the grades and scores may be tempted to assume that the test taker just had a bad day while taking the test, and may discount the low test score in favor of the high grades. But if the test is retaken and the scores are approximately the same, then the validity of the low scores are only confirmed. Therefore, a retake could actually hurt a test taker by definitely bracketing a test taker's score ability to a limited range.